ATLAS OF
TRANSNASAL ESOPHAGOSCOPY

ATLAS OF
TRANSNASAL
ESOPHAGOSCOPY

Gregory N. Postma, MD

Professor
Department of Otolaryngology
Director, Center for Voice and Swallowing Disorders
Medical College of Georgia
Augusta, Georgia

Peter C. Belafsky, MD, PhD

Assistant Professor and Medical Director
Center for Voice and Swallowing
Department of Otolaryngology/Head and Neck Surgery
University of California Davis School of Medicine
Sacramento, California

Jonathan E. Aviv, MD

Professor of Otolaryngology/Head and Neck Surgery and Medical Director
Voice and Swallowing Center
Department of Otolaryngology
College of Physicians and Surgeons
Columbia University
New York Presbyterian Hospital
New York, New York

With Foreword by Jamie A. Koufman, MD

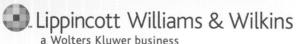

Lippincott Williams & Wilkins
a Wolters Kluwer business

Philadelphia • Baltimore • New York • London
Buenos Aires • Hong Kong • Sydney • Tokyo

Acquisitions Editor: Robert Hurley/Susan Rhyner
Managing Editor: Michelle LaPlante
Project Manager: Nicole Walz
Manufacturing Coordinator: Kathleen Brown
Marketing Manager: Angela Panetta
Interior Designer: Stephen Druding
Cover Designer: Joseph DePinho
Production Services: Maryland Composition Co., Inc.
Printer: RR Donnelley-China

Printed in China

Library of Congress Cataloging-in-Publication Data

Postma, Gregory N.
    Atlas of transnasal esophagoscopy / Gregory N. Postma, Peter C. Belafsky, Jonathan E. Aviv.
        p. ; cm.
    Includes bibliographical references.
    ISBN 0-7817-5180-2
1. Esophagoscopy—Atlases. I. Belafsky, Peter C. II. Aviv, Jonathan E., 1960- III. Title.
    [DNLM: 1. Esophagoscopy—methods—Atlases.   2. Esophageal Diseases—diagnosis—Atlases.
3. Esophageal Diseases—therapy—Atlases. WI 17 P858a 2006]
RC815.7.P67 2006
616.3'200223—dc22

                                                                                2006004708

TABLE OF CONTENTS

Preface   *vii*
Acknowledgments   *ix*
Foreword   *xi*

1	**Indications for Transnasal Esophagoscopy**	*1*
2	**Technique and Endoscopic Anatomy of Nasal Cavity and Hypopharynx**	*5*
3	**Normal Transnasal Esophagoscopy**	*17*
4	**Esophagitis**	*25*
5	**Webs and Rings**	*37*
6	**Hiatal Hernia**	*43*
7	**Barrett's Metaplasia**	*51*
8	**Neoplasia**	*59*
9	**Miscellaneous Esophageal Disorders**	*69*
10	**Procedures**	*89*

Index   *103*

PREFACE

Transnasal esophagoscopy (TNE) has significantly altered the clinical practices of endoscopists from various disciplines. In just a short time, it has transformed the way clinicians evaluate the esophagus and it has been the stimulus for dozens of hands-on courses each year, teaching otolaryngologists, gastroenterologists, and laparoscopic surgeons how to perform TNE and how to incorporate it into their offices.

Atlas of Transnasal Esophagoscopy is a concise yet comprehensive review of TNE, and it is our hope that this work will assist both novice and experienced examiners in understanding esophageal disease and the various uses of TNE. Determining which patients will benefit from TNE is a key question, and so we begin with four indications. We then describe the technique of TNE and provide a review of nasal, laryngopharyngeal, and endoscopic esophageal anatomy.

The next six chapters are devoted to various types of esophageal pathology including, but not limited to, various causes of esophagitis, webs and rings, hiatal hernias, Barrett's esophagus, and esophageal neoplasia. Each area of pathology will briefly note treatment options to assist the physician in determining the need for immediate therapy or further specialist consultation.

Finally, this exciting technology enables the endoscopist to perform a number of other in-office procedures. These procedures are reviewed and references are provided for detailed descriptions.

It is our belief that this atlas will serve as a valuable resource for otolaryngologists, gastroenterologists, general and laparoscopic surgeons, as well as others interested in esophagoscopy at any level of training and experience. I would encourage the readers of this atlas to contact any of the authors to discuss clinical dilemmas involving their patients and to provide us with any ideas on how we may improve further editions of this book.

Gregory N. Postma, MD
Center for Voice and Swallowing Disorders
Professor, Department of Otolaryngology
Medical College of Georgia
Augusta, GA 30912-4060
gpostma@mcg.edu

ACKNOWLEDGMENTS

All of the authors are in debt to Dr. Larry Johnson, whose experience, insight, advice, and friendship have contributed greatly to our knowledge of esophagology and made the publication of this atlas possible.

In particular, I wish to recognize and thank Dr. Jamie Koufman, Dr. Jonathan Aviv, and Dr. Reza Shaker for their vision and leadership roles in the development and popularizing of the unsedated transnasal evaluation of the upper aerodigestive tract.

I would also like to acknowledge and thank Dr. Jamie A. Koufman of Wake Forest University, Dr. Mark Belafsky, Dr. Milan Amin of New York University, and Dr. Timothy Anderson of Boston Medical Center, as well as all of the authors who supplied clinical images for this atlas.

—**Gregory N. Postma, MD**

FOREWORD

Since the early 1900s and the era of Chevalier Jackson, the esophagus has been within the domain of the otolaryngologist. Early instruments were large-bore, rigid endoscopes that required some form of anesthesia for their use. For most of the 20th century, the most common indications for esophagoscopy were diagnostic and for foreign body retrieval. Since the introduction of the fiberoptic esophagoscope in the 1960s, gastroenterologists have been performing diagnostic and interventional esophagoscopy.

In 2000, the distal-chip camera esophagoscope was introduced to our field by Pentax. Since that time, its otolaryngologic applications have grown exponentially. The optics are spectacular, and the external diameter is small enough to be comfortably introduced transnasally. In addition, there is a 2-mm working channel that allows irrigation, air insufflation, biopsy, and the performance of a variety of procedures.

The transnasal esophagoscope is now being used for panendoscopy and multiple new applications in the esophagus, laryngopharynx, and tracheobronchial tree. In addition, when coupled to pulsed-dye, carbon dioxide, or thalium:YAG lasers, this technology has allowed for the proliferation of safe and effective, unsedated, in-office laryngeal surgery.

The shift to office-based procedures that is occurring in otolaryngology is a function of not only advances in technology, but also of advances in clinical medicine and concerns about healthcare costs. As more is known about laryngopharyngeal reflux and Barrett's esophagus, more and more patients with hoarseness, globus, dysphagia, and chronic cough will benefit from unsedated, in-office endoscopy.

The further development of minimally invasive endoscopy for the diagnosis and treatment of aerodigestive tract disorders will continue to advance bronchoesophagology. We hope that this book will help both the otolaryngologist and gastroenterologist move forward into this exciting new world.

Jamie A. Koufman, MD, FACS, Director
Center for Voice and Swallowing Disorders
Wake Forest University
Professor of Surgery (Otolaryngology)
Wake Forest University School of Medicine
Wake Forest University Baptist Medical Center
Medical Center Boulevard
Winston-Salem, NC

1

Indications for Transnasal Esophagoscopy

The indications for transnasal esophagoscopy (TNE) can be divided into two main categories: those with esophageal and those with extraesophageal requirements for the procedure. These indications can be further subclassified into diagnostic and therapeutic categories. The relative esophageal indications established by the American Society for Gastrointestinal Endoscopy (ASGE) and the American College of Gastroenterology (ACG) are summarized in Table 1.1 (1,2). Warning signs necessitating early endoscopy include dysphagia, bleeding, choking, chest pain, and weight loss (1). Although the ASGE indications predict endoscopic findings and serve as a useful benchmark, significant endoscopic diagnoses have been reported in up to 28% of endoscopies that did not meet ASGE criteria (3). Strict adherence to these guidelines can miss important pathology, and the ultimate decision to perform endoscopy must be tailored to the individual clinical scenario.

Although the extraesophageal indications for TNE are still being defined, relative indications include globus pharyngeus, chronic cough, cervical dysphagia, head and neck cancer, poorly controlled asthma, odynophagia, hemoptysis, and moderate to severe laryngopharyngeal reflux (Table 1.2). A certain cohort of individuals with globus, dysphagia, chronic cough, and odynophagia unresponsive to traditional therapy may have alternative pathology in their esophagus responsible for their symptoms. Our experience with TNE in persons with chronic cough

---

TABLE 1.1
Relative Esophageal Indications for TNE

Diagnostic
- Esophageal symptoms that persist despite an appropriate trial of therapy
- Dysphagia
- Odynophagia
- Weight loss
- Anorexia
- For evaluation of radiologically demonstrated lesions
- To assess acute injury after caustic ingestion
- Longstanding symptoms of gastroesophageal reflux disease (5 yr)
- Persons requiring continuous antireflux therapy
- Foreign body evaluation and possible removal
- Portal hypertension or cirrhosis to screen for or evaluate varices
- Passage of guide wire for placement of manometry catheter in severe achalasia

Therapeutic
- Dilation of strictures
- Placement of feeding tubes under direct vision
- Treatment of achalasia (botulinum toxin type A)
- Endoscopic laser therapy
- Placement of wireless pH telemetry capsule

> **TABLE 1.2**
> Relative Extraesophageal Indications for TNE
>
> - Globus pharyngeus
> - Chronic cough
> - Cervical dysphagia
> - Poorly controlled asthma or chronic obstructive pulmonary disease
> - Odynophagia
> - Hemoptysis
> - Laryngopharyngeal reflux
> - Head and neck cancer

suggests that these individuals suffer from more severe esophageal inflammatory disease and are possibly at a higher risk for Barrett's metaplasia, even in the absence of heartburn. Although the risk of Barrett's metaplasia in these individuals has not been adequately described, we routinely screen the esophagus of all individuals with chronic cough. The indications for TNE in patients with laryngopharyngeal reflux (LPR) are more controversial. The prevalence of Barrett's metaplasia in persons with LPR has been reported to be 7% (4). This does not appear to be different from the prevalence of Barrett's metaplasia among volunteers undergoing colonoscopy (5). These data suggest that TNE for persons with mild LPR is probably not indicated. Reavis et al., however, reported that symptoms of LPR were significantly more prevalent than typical gastroesophageal reflux symptoms in persons with adenocarcinoma or dysplasia of the esophagus (6). Their data suggest that symptoms of LPR may be the only indication of esophageal metaplasia or malignancy. LPR patients who respond to reflux therapy may have underlying esophageal pathology that becomes masked once antireflux treatment is initiated. Missing underlying esophageal metaplasia, dysplasia, or carcinoma in patients with LPR could have devastating consequences. Thus, until the indications for TNE in persons with LPR can be better defined, screening individuals with this disorder is reasonable, particularly if they have other risk factors. This practice will likely detect some patients with early esophageal adenocarcinoma or dysplasia whom otherwise would not have their esophagus examined.

REFERENCES

1. DeVault KR, Castell DO. Updated guidelines for the diagnosis and treatment of gastroesophageal reflux disease. The Practice Parameters Committee of the American College of Gastroenterology. *Am J Gastroenterol* 1999;94(6):1434–1442.
2. American Society for Gastrointestinal Endoscopy. Appropriate use of gastrointestinal endoscopy. *Gastrointest Endosc* 2000;52:831–837.
3. Schenk BE, Kuipers EJ, Klinkenberg-Knol EC, et al. Omeprazole as a diagnostic tool in gastroesophageal reflux disease. *Am J Gastroenterol* 1997;92:1997–2000.

4. Koufman JA, Belafsky PC, Bach KK, et al. Prevalence of esophagitis in patients with pH-documented laryngopharyngeal reflux. *Laryngoscope* 2002;112(9):1606–1609.

5. Rex DK, Cummings OW, Shaw M, et al. Screening for Barrett's esophagus in colonoscopy patients with and without heartburn. *Gastroenterology* 2003;125(6):1670–1677.

6. Reavis KM, Morris CD, Gopal DV, et al. Laryngopharyngeal reflux symptoms better predict the presence of esophageal adenocarcinoma than typical gastroesophageal reflux symptoms. *Ann Surg* 2004;239(6):849–856; discussion 856–858.

2

Technique and Endoscopic Anatomy of Nasal Cavity and Hypopharynx

INTRODUCTION

Transnasal esophagoscopy (TNE) is performed by placing a small-caliber, flexible endoscope via the nose into the hypopharynx and then into the esophagus. TNE is performed with the patient awake, sitting upright in a chair. No conscious, or intravenous, sedation is used (1–5). The key to successful performance of TNE is adequate topical anesthesia and vasoconstriction in the nasal cavity (Fig. 2.1). Before the technique of TNE is addressed in detail, a review of basic endoscopic anatomy of the nasal cavity and hypopharynx will be given. Examples of common nasal and hypopharyngeal pathology will be shown to familiarize the endoscopist with several variations of the endoscopic anatomy that may be encountered as the esophagoscope is passed from the nostril into the esophagus.

In contrast with transoral esophagogastroduodenoscopy (EGD), the image orientation on the video monitor is such that the tongue base is at the superior portion of the monitor (i.e., at 12 o'clock), and the esophageal inlet is located inferior to the tongue base. During TNE, the tongue base and esophageal inlet are consistently in the anatomic position familiar to most otolaryngologists, with the base of tongue located at the inferior portion of the monitor (i.e., at 6 o'clock) with the esophageal inlet superior to the tongue base and "behind" the arytenoid cartilages (i.e., at 12 o'clock) (Fig. 2.2).

Nasal Anatomy

The TNE scope should be placed in the side of the nasal cavity that is most patent. Therefore, a nasal examination is performed prior to TNE to determine the less obstructed side. Three primary structures in the nose have to be visualized to ensure safe, unobstructed passage: the nasal septum and the inferior and middle turbinates (Fig. 2.3). There are two ways of passing

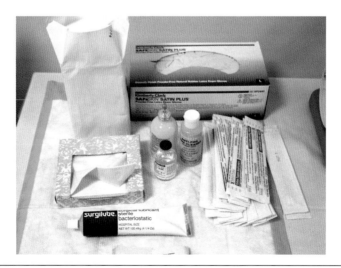

Figure 2.1 ● Materials necessary for administration of anesthesia prior to transnasal esophagoscopy. A bottle of Xylocaine 1% with epinephrine 1:100,000 for spray or application with cotton-tipped applicators, a bottle of benzocaine 20%, Surgilube or Xylocaine jelly, and a defogging solution may be used. Other topical anesthetics and decongestants work equally well.

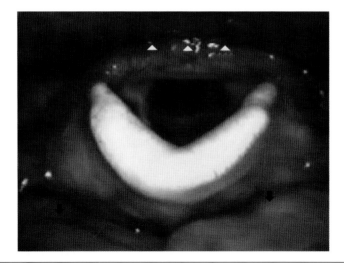

Figure 2.2 ● Endoscopic orientation of hypopharynx during transnasal esophagoscopy.
The tongue base (*black arrows*) is inferior and the esophageal inlet (*white arrowheads*) is at the superior portion of the image.

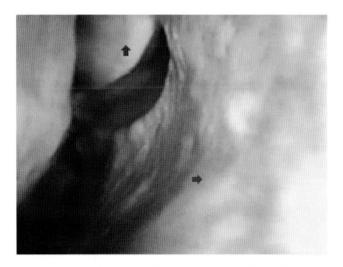

Figure 2.3 ● Endoscopic view of right nasal cavity.   Note the nasal septum (*red arrow*), middle turbinate (*blue arrow*), and inferior turbinate (*green arrow*). There is a slight nasal septal spur posteriorly (*red arrow*).

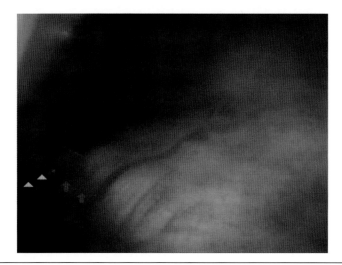

Figure 2.4 ● Endoscopic view of a right nasal cavity.   Note that the deviated nasal septum (*red arrows*) is touching the inferior turbinate (*blue arrowheads*), causing near complete nasal obstruction.

the scope through the nose. One is to pass the scope between the middle and inferior turbinates, and the other option is to pass the scope along the floor of the nose, usually inferior and medial to the inferior turbinate. The majority of the time, the authors prefer the latter route.

Certain variations in normal anatomy may make transnasal passage of the scope difficult. Nasal septal deviations are a very common cause of unilateral nasal obstruction (Fig. 2.4). Generally, if one side of the nose has a markedly deviated septum, the other side is more patent and will allow easier passage of the endoscope. Another relatively common variation, and one that can be confusing to the endoscopist, is a nasal septal perforation (Fig. 2.5). Care must be

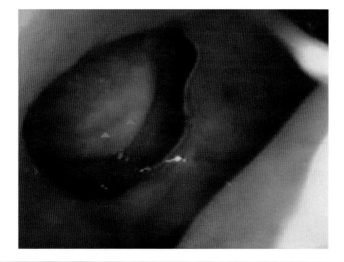

Figure 2.5 ● Endoscopic view of a nasal septal perforation.   View is from the left nasal cavity; the *right* middle turbinate (*blue arrowheads*) is seen through the septal perforation (*red arrowheads*).

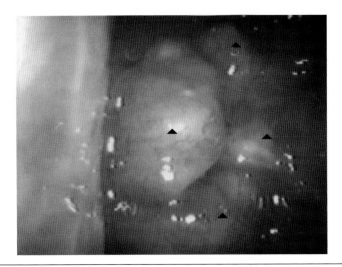

Figure 2.6 ● Nasal polyps (*arrowheads*). The polypoid mass is occupying the entire right nasal cavity. The right inferior turbinate is visualized just anterior to the polyps.

taken not to inadvertently traverse or traumatize the opening in the perforated septum as such a maneuver will likely make it difficult to readily advance the scope, as well as possibly causing septal trauma and epistaxis. Another common pathological condition of the nasal cavity are nasal polyps, which can cause significant nasal obstruction (Fig. 2.6). When nasal polyps are seen, it is preferable to pass the scope on the side where the polyps are smallest. If the endoscope cannot be passed through either nostril, then a standard gastrointestinal oral endoscopy appliance can be used to pass the scope transorally (Fig. 2.7). More topical anesthesia on the tongue base is needed to perform unsedated per-oral esophagoscopy.

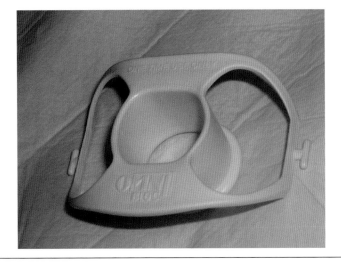

Figure 2.7 ● An oral appliance placed in the patient's mouth to enable safe passage of the transnasal esophagoscope in individuals with severe nasal obstruction.

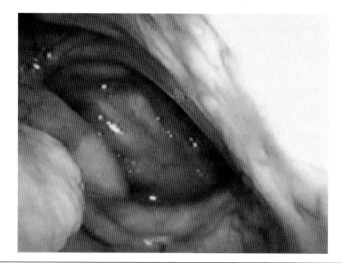

Figure 2.8 ● Endoscopic view of nasopharynx and torus tubarius. The view is from the right nasal cavity, and the torus is located at 9 o'clock. The nasopharynx is medial to the torus.

Once the nasal cavity is traversed, attention is directed toward the nasopharynx. The torus tubarius is the anatomic landmark representing the eustachian tube opening into the nasopharynx (Fig. 2.8). After the scope is passed through the nasopharynx, the base of tongue, vallecula, and supraglottic structures are encountered. A detailed endoscopic inspection and digital palpation of the tongue base and vallecula in persons with dysphagia are necessary to exclude pathology in this region (Fig. 2.9).

After tongue base inspection, the larynx is visualized. Attention should be focused on the presence or absence of laryngeal lesions (Fig. 2.10). In addition, vocal fold motion abnormali-

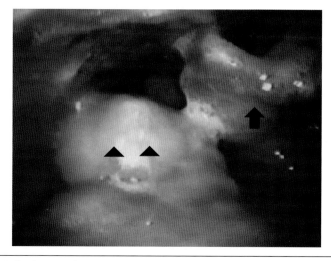

Figure 2.9 ● Right base of tongue tumor (*arrowheads*). An oval mass can be seen in the vallecula with the lingual aspect of the epiglottis in the background (*arrow*).

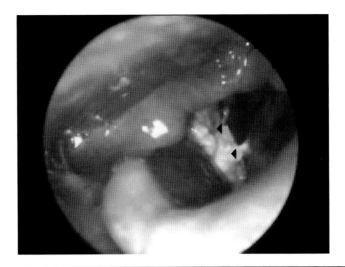

Figure 2.10 ● Right vocal fold squamous cell carcinoma (*arrowheads*).

ties (paralysis or paresis) should be sought. Vocal fold immobility in a person with dysphagia could be caused by a neoplasm in the skull base, neck, or mediastinum (Fig. 2.11).

TNE Technique

Although not absolutely necessary, it is preferable that the patient not eat or drink for at least 3 hours before TNE. This ensures that the stomach is empty during the examination. No conscious, or intravenous, sedation is used. The key to successful examination is adequate topical nasal anesthesia and decongestion. While a standard per-oral gastroscope is approximately

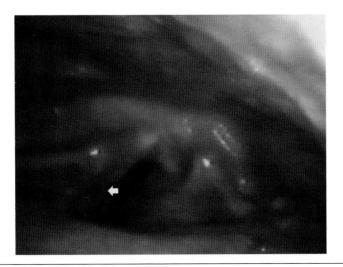

Figure 2.11 ● Right vocal fold paralysis. Note that left true vocal fold is widely abducted (*arrow*) but that the right true vocal fold is in the paramedian position.

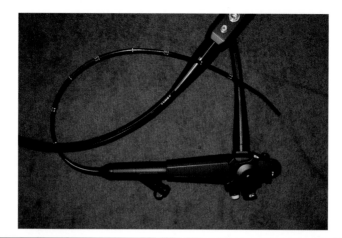

Figure 2.12 ● Video chip transnasal esophagoscope. The chip camera is built into the distal tip of the endoscope.

10 to 12 mm in diameter, the transnasal esophagoscope ranges in diameter from 4.5 to 5.1 mm. There are two different types of TNE systems available. One is a video chip flexible endoscope system where the camera is located on the distal tip of the endoscope and the scope is attached to a video processor (Fig. 2.12). The other is an add-on camera flexible endoscope system in which a camera is attached to the proximal portion of the fiberscope, usually at the eyepiece (Fig. 2.13). The fiberoptic add-on camera system can incorporate a single-use, disposable TNE EndoSheath (Fig. 2.14). The distal chip endoscopes and endo sheaths have a channel for air

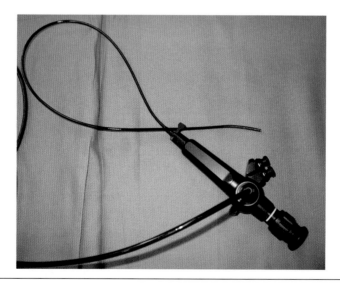

Figure 2.13 ● Fiberoptic add-on camera transnasal esophagoscope. The camera is placed on the proximal end of the scope, where the eyepiece is located.

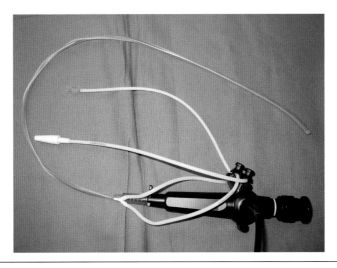

Figure 2.14 ● **Add-on camera transnasal esophagoscope with EndoSheath.**   There are two pinch valves on the scope: one that allows for air insufflation and one that allows for suction.

insufflation or water instillation and for suction. A working channel allowing passage of a 1.8–mm cup forceps, biopsy brushes, or flexible lasers is also available (Fig. 2.15).

The patient's nasal cavity is anesthetized and vasoconstricted with a topical agent, typically lidocaine 1% to 2% with epinephrine 1:100,000 or oxymetazoline 0.05%. The hypopharynx may be lightly anesthetized with benzocaine 20% spray administered via the oral cavity. Too much hypopharyngeal anesthesia actually makes TNE more difficult, as patient secretions accumulate in the hypopharynx, penetrate the larynx, and cause the patient to aspirate and cough.

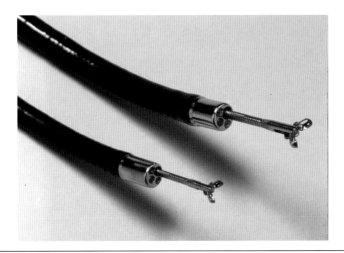

Figure 2.15 ● **Biopsy forceps emerging from video chip transnasal esophagoscopes.**

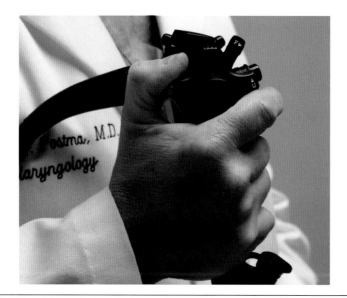

Figure 2.16 ● **Holding the endoscope** in a more vertical fashion similar to the gastroenterologist technique.

The esophagoscope can be held in various ways. The two most common are the "standard" manner similar to gastroenterologists (Fig. 2.16) and the "fishing pole" technique (Fig. 2.17). Each examiner should determine which is most effective for him- or herself.

The lubricated endoscope is then inserted through the nose and, depending on the patient, the TNE is inserted into the esophagus using two different techniques. In one technique, the patient is asked to eructate. During the burp, the cricopharyngeus opens and the endoscope

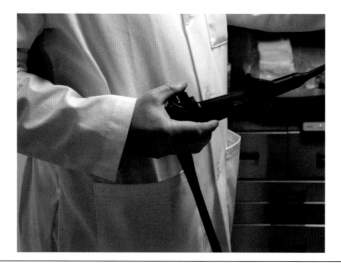

Figure 2.17 ● **The "fishing pole" technique of transnasal esophagoscopy.**

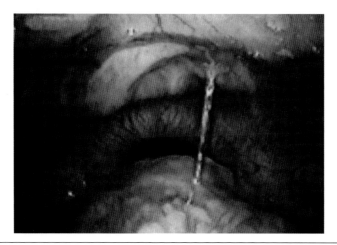

Figure 2.18 ● Endoscopic view of cricopharyngeal opening just prior to esophageal intubation with the transnasal esophagoscope.

can be passed posterior to the cricoid into the cervical esophagus (Fig. 2.18). The other technique, which is more commonly used, is to have the patient tuck their chin toward their chest and then swallow. The endoscope tip is just above the arytenoids or in the left pyriform sinus. One should provide gentle pressure on the postcricoid region with the endoscope during the initiation of the swallow. As the laryngohyoid complex moves superiorly and anteriorly, the upper esophageal sphincter (UES) opens and the esophagus is intubated. Difficulty in traversing the UES may indicate the presence of a Zenker's diverticulum or a hypertonic cricopharyngeus muscle. If excessive resistance is encountered, the procedure should be terminated, and a barium swallow or modified barium swallow (depending on the clinical scenario) should be obtained to further evaluate the hypopharynx and cervical esophagus.

Once the esophagus is entered, the endoscope is passed to the region of the squamocolumnar junction (SCJ) and lower esophageal sphincter (LES). The middle and proximal esophagus is examined in greater detail during withdrawal of the endoscope. The SCJ is visualized, and the presence of pathology in this region is evaluated. Having the patient swallow during this portion of the examination will open the LES and help visualize the terminal linear blood vessels and the SCJ. Sniffing will narrow the diaphragmatic hiatus and assist the examiner in evaluating the anatomy of this complex region. If necessary, a biopsy is obtained. The authors do not typically biopsy normal-appearing mucosa. The endoscope is then passed deeper into the stomach, and a retroflexed view of the LES is obtained. This maneuver is performed by insufflating more air into the stomach and deflecting the tip of the endoscope into a "U" shape by counter-clockwise rotation of the control wheel. The endoscope is then twisted 90 to 180 degrees in order to bring the endoscope shaft into view. After examining the esophagogastric junction and gastric cardia from below, the stomach is then suctioned free of air, and the esophagoscope is straightened and gently withdrawn. Failure to suction air out of the stomach can result in severe belching and vomiting on occasion. A combination of air insufflation and suction is necessary to keep the patient comfortable, the esophagus distended, and the tip of the endoscope clean. Every millimeter of esophageal mucosa is visualized during removal of the endoscope. The postcricoid area is visualized by generous air insufflation as the endoscope is removed from the esophagus and the videotape can then be reviewed, since often only a few frames of this region are obtained.

Patient Acceptance and Toleration

A series of 700 consecutive patients undergoing TNE was recently reported and was well tolerated by 98% of individuals (6). This is in contrast to the experience at some gastroenterology centers (7–9). This ready acceptance of TNE by patients in otolaryngologic practices may be due to various factors. The first is the gastroenterology patients' expectation that they will feel or remember nothing from the procedure itself. It is difficult at times to suggest to a patient with such a preconception to pursue an unsedated examination. The other reason is that the vast majority of otolaryngology patients have already undergone a flexible endoscopic examination of their larynx and pharynx. So they have already experienced a major portion of the endoscopy, and it also allows the endoscopist to select a cooperative patient for TNE. In other words, if a patient did not tolerate the laryngeal examination, it would make little sense to attempt to perform TNE.

REFERENCES

1. Aviv JE, Takoudes T, Ma G, et al. Office-based esophagoscopy: a preliminary report. *Otolaryngol Head Neck Surg* 2001;125:170–175.
2. Belafsky PC. Office endoscopy for the laryngologist/bronchoesophagologist. *Curr Opin Otolaryngol Head Neck Surg* 2002;10:467–471.
3. Belafsky PC, Postma GN, Daniels E, et al. Transnasal esophagoscopy. *Otolaryngol Head Neck Surg* 2001;125:588–589.
4. Postma GN, Amin MR, Simpson CB, et al. Office procedures for the esophagus. *Ear Nose Throat J* 2004;83(7 Suppl 2):17–21.
5. Andrus JG, Dolan RW, Anderson TD. Transnasal esophagoscopy: a high-yield diagnostic tool. *Laryngoscope* 2005;115(6):993–996.
6. Postma, GN, Cohen JT, Belafsky PC, et al. Transnasal esophagoscopy: revisited (over 700 consecutive cases). *Laryngoscope* 2005;115(2):321–323.
7. Thota PN, Zuccaro G Jr, Vargo JJ 2nd, et al. A randomized prospective trial comparing unsedated esophagoscopy via transnasal and transoral routes using a 4-mm video endoscope with conventional endoscopy with sedation. *Endoscopy* 2005;37:559–565.
8. Faulx AL, Catanzaro A, Zyzanski S, et al. Patient tolerance and acceptance of unsedated ultrathin esophagoscopy. *Gastrointest Endosc* 2002;55:620–623.
9. L. Johnson, personal communication, 2005.

3

Normal Transnasal Esophagoscopy

The esophagus is a muscular tube that originates in the pharynx and terminates in the stomach. It begins at the level of the 6th cervical vertebrae at the lower end of the cricoid cartilage and averages 20 to 22 cm in length. It traverses the diaphragmatic hiatus at the level of the 10th thoracic vertebrae and ends at the cardia of the stomach at the 11th thoracic vertebrae. The esophageal wall consists of both skeletal and smooth muscle. Striated muscle makes up approximately 5% of the wall of the proximal esophagus. The midesophagus (35%–40%) has a wall of mixed striated and smooth muscle, and the distal 50% to 60% of the esophageal wall is made up of smooth muscle fibers. There is no serosal layer.

The upper esophageal sphincter (UES) is a 2- to 4-cm high-pressure zone which is usually the narrowest portion of the esophagus. It is primarily made up by the cricopharyngeus muscle, which is tonically contracted at rest.

The lower esophageal sphincter (LES) is both anatomic and physiologic. It contains muscle fibers from both the esophagus and diaphragm. The sphincter is thickest on the greater curvature of the stomach and averages 31 mm in length. The fibers are not complete rings but form semicircles and terminate along the anterior and posterior walls of the stomach. The distance to the LES from the nasal ala is approximately 41 cm.

The esophagus is lined by squamous epithelium. At the distal esophagus, the mucosa changes to gastric columnar epithelium. This junction is called the squamocolumnar junction (SCJ), the ora serrata, or the Z-line (Fig. 3.1).

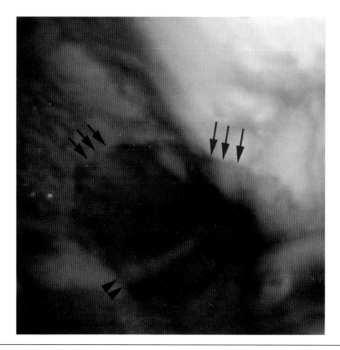

Figure 3.1 ● Normal squamocolumnar junction (*blue arrows*). The termination of the linear esophageal mucosal vessels from above (*black arrows*) and the gastric rugae from below (*black arrowheads*) delineate the gastroesophageal junction (GEJ) .

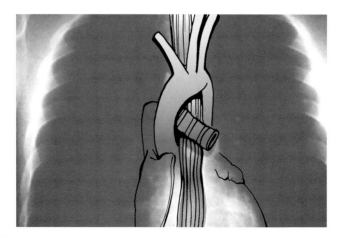

Figure 3.2 ● The three external compressions of the esophagus, from superior to inferior: the aortic, left main-stem bronchus, and diaphragmatic compressions.

The anatomy of the esophagus as visualized through the thin transnasal esophagoscope is different from that seen through the transoral endoscope, and is also different from that seen with the rigid esophagoscope. The thin transnasal endoscopes do not distort the normal anatomical relationships, and this allows the normal sphincters, curves, and extrinsic compressions to be easily visualized. The patient is upright in the anatomical position so that left/right and anterior/posterior can easily be discerned on the monitor.

The esophagus starts in the midline and deviates three times before it enters the gastric cardia. The first curve is to the left at the base of the neck. It then curves gently back to the midline at approximately T5. The next curve is to the left again at T7. The final curve is distal, where the esophagus curves anteriorly to pass through the diaphragm. There is also a gentle anterior-posterior curve as the esophagus descends adjacent to the bony spinal column. There are three primary external compressions. From superior to inferior, they are the aortic, left main bronchus, and diaphragmatic compressions (Fig. 3.2). The aortic compression is a pulsatile compression on the left anterior-lateral wall at approximately 24 cm from the nasal ala (Fig. 3.3). The left mainstem bronchus produces an anterior compression at approximately 26 cm from the nasal ala (Fig. 3.4). The diaphragmatic compression occurs at the distal esophagus and produces a lateral and medial constriction (Fig. 3.5). It is best visualized by having the patient perform a sniffing maneuver that opens and closes the diaphragm so that it may be localized.

The squamous mucosa lining the esophagus appears universally whitish-pale. A fine network of terminal linear vessels can be seen in the distal third of the esophagus and terminates at the gastric rugae. These do not normally extend below the SCJ. Four to five folds of gastric mucosa (rugae) form longitudinal folds at or just below the gastroesophageal junction (GEJ). The termination of the linear esophageal mucosal vessels from above and the gastric rugae from below provide useful landmarks to identify the GEJ (Fig. 3.1).

The normal SCJ is circular in nature. An irregular Z-line, however, is not necessarily pathologic (Fig. 3.6). The squamocolumnar transition zone should occur where the network

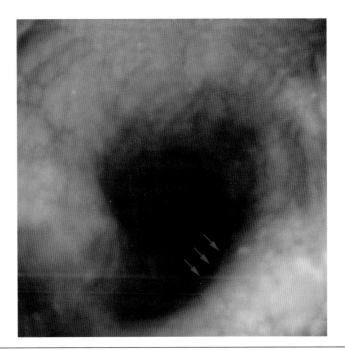

Figure 3.3 ● **Endoscopic image of the aortic compression 24 cm from the nasal ala.**
Note that the compression is left anterolateral (*blue arrows*).

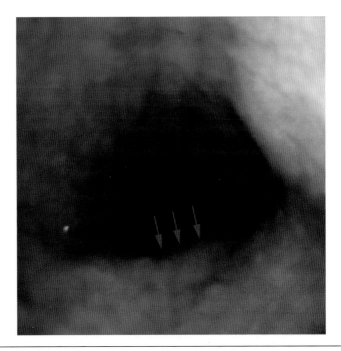

Figure 3.4 ● **Endoscopic image of the left mainstem bronchus compression 26 cm from the nasal ala.** Note that the compression is anterior (*blue arrows*).

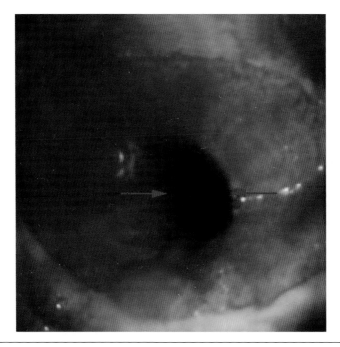

Figure 3.5 ● Endoscopic image of the diaphragmatic compression 41 cm from the nasal ala. Note that the compression is lateral and medial (*blue arrows*).

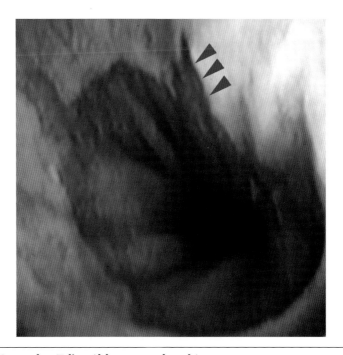

Figure 3.6 ● Irregular Z-line (*blue arrowheads*).

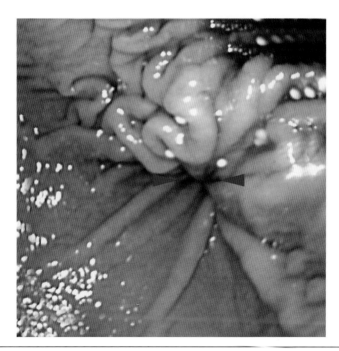

Figure 3.7 ● Extension of gastric rugae 3.5 cm above diaphragmatic hiatus (*blue arrowheads*), indicating a hiatal hernia.

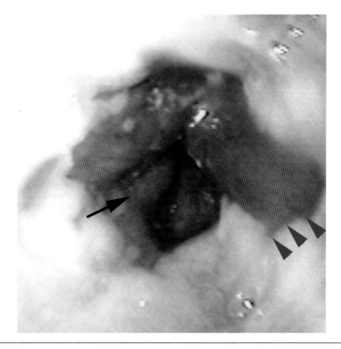

Figure 3.8 ● A 2-cm tongue of short-segment Barrett's metaplasia (*blue arrowheads*).
The esophageal mucosa is edematous, indicating the presence of esophagitis. The GEJ is difficult to identify because the squamocolumnar junction is in an abnormal location secondary to the Barrett's metaplasia. The linear esophageal mucosal vessels are concealed by the edematous mucosa that further complicates delineation of the true GEJ. The location of the GEJ is estimated by the location of the gastric rugae (black arrow).

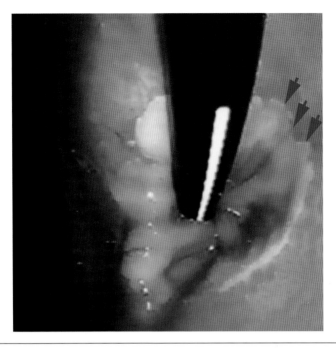

Figure 3.9 ● **Normal retroverted view of squamocolumnar junction (*blue arrows*).** Note that the hiatus is tight around the endoscope.

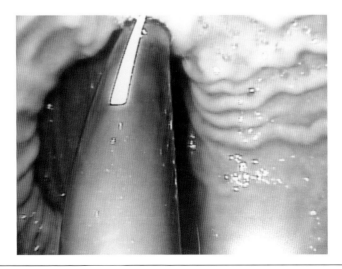

Figure 3.10 ● **Retroflexed view of a sliding hiatal hernia.**

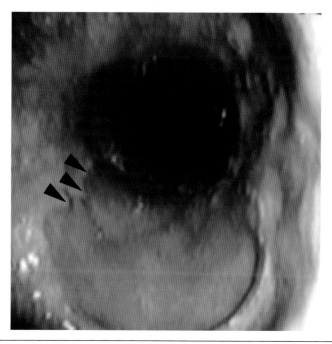

Figure 3.11 ● **Heterotopic gastric epithelium in the cervical esophagus (inlet patch).**

of esophageal vessels terminate and the gastric rugae begin. The gastric rugae may be seen to extend 1 to 2 cm above the compression of the diaphragmatic hiatus. Any proximal extension of the rugae 2 cm above the hiatus would be indicative of a hiatal hernia (Fig. 3.7). Any migration of gastric-appearing mucosa above the GEJ into the esophageal mucosa would suggest the presence of Barrett's metaplasia (Fig. 3.8). Upon retroflexion, the hiatus should be tight around the endoscope (Fig. 3.9). A lax diaphragmatic crus seen during retroflexion view is indicative of a hiatal hernia (Fig. 3.10).

Occasionally, a small patch of heterotopic gastric mucosa can be seen in the cervical esophagus (Fig. 3.11). This inlet patch may secrete acid but is usually of no clinical significance.

4

Esophagitis

INTRODUCTION

Esophagitis is one of the most common findings encountered during transnasal esophagoscopy (TNE). It has several etiologies, including acid reflux, foreign bodies (e.g., pills), infection, allergy, caustic injury, as well as a sequela of radiation therapy.

REFLUX ESOPHAGITIS

The ability to consistently describe the endoscopic findings in a patient with suspected reflux esophagitis is important. Although there are several grading systems for esophagitis, the Los Angeles (LA) classification system is the most widely accepted (1). The LA classification system is based on the extent of esophageal mucosal breaks seen endoscopically. A mucosal break is defined as an area of slough or an area of erythema with a discrete line of demarcation from the adjacent or normal-looking mucosa. The mucosal breaks are then classified by a grading scale: A, B, C, and D (2). The reference point used in determining the extent of the mucosal break is the peak of the mucosal folds in the esophagus, best seen during partial air insufflation of the esophagus. In grade A esophagitis, the mucosal breaks are less than 5 mm in length and do not extend between the tops of two esophageal mucosal folds (Fig. 4.1). With grade B esophagitis, the mucosal breaks are longer than 5 mm, but confined to the mucosal fold of the esophagus, so that they are not contiguous between the tops of the two mucosal folds (Fig. 4.2). In grade C esophagitis, the mucosal breaks are continuous between the tops of two or more mucosal folds but less than 75% of the esophageal circumference (Fig. 4.3). In grade D esophagitis, the mucosal break involves at least 75% of the circumference of the esophagus (Fig. 4.4). As esophagitis becomes more severe, complications of esophagitis may ensue, such as stricture. An esophageal stricture is defined as a circumferential narrowing of the esophagus (Fig. 4.5).

CANDIDA ESOPHAGITIS

Esophagitis caused by *Candida albicans* is the most common infectious cause of esophagitis (3). The most commonly reported symptoms are odynophagia and dysphagia, though up to 25% of patients can be asymptomatic (4). Some individuals, however, will present with symptoms suggestive of laryngopharyngeal reflux such as globus, excessive throat clearing, or excessive mucous. Risk factors for the development of *Candida* esophagitis include the presence of HIV infection, postradiation or chemotherapy, diabetes mellitus, steroid use, and diseases of impaired esophageal peristalsis such as progressive systemic sclerosis (scleroderma). It is important to note that a normal flexible laryngoscopy and oropharyngeal examination do not eliminate the possibility of fungal esophagitis. We have seen dozens of patients who are immunocompetent and not using steroids with *Candida* esophagitis and no significant physical findings in the laryngopharynx.

The endoscopic appearance of *Candida* esophagitis is characterized by mucosal plaques, often punctate, typically yellow to tan (Fig. 4.6). As the disease increases in severity, the scattered mucosal plaques begin to coalesce, ultimately resulting in a circumferential coating

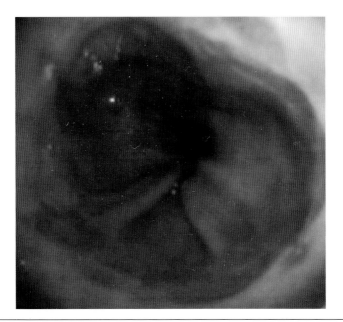

Figure 4.1 ● Grade A esophagitis. The mucosal breaks are less than 5 mm in length and do not extend between the tops of two mucosal folds.

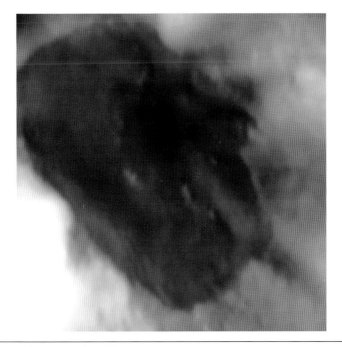

Figure 4.2 ● Grade B esophagitis. The mucosal breaks longer than 5 mm are confined to the mucosal fold, i.e., not contiguous between the tops of the two mucosal folds.

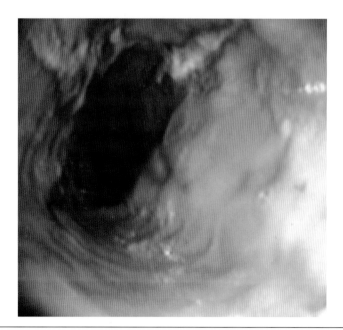

Figure 4.3 ● Grade C esophagitis.   The mucosal breaks are continuous between the tops of two or more mucosal folds, but less than 75% of the esophageal circumference.

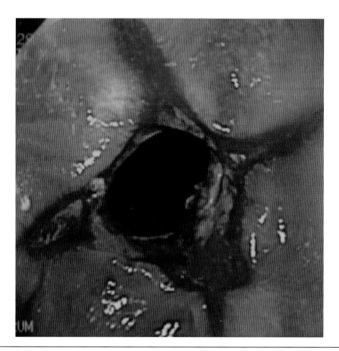

Figure 4.4 ● Grade D esophagitis.   The mucosal break involves at least 75% of the circumference of the esophagus.

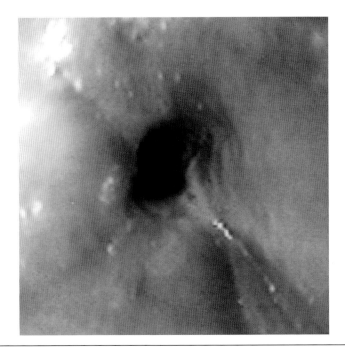

Figure 4.5 ● Esophageal stricture.   There is circumferential narrowing of the esophagus.

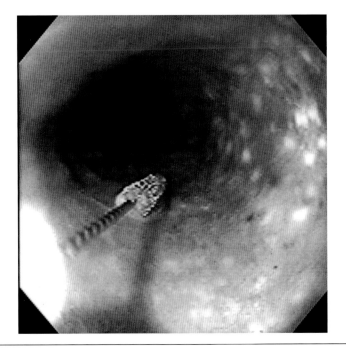

Figure 4.6 ● *Candida* esophagitis.   Isolated yellow, tan plaques line the esophageal mucosa.

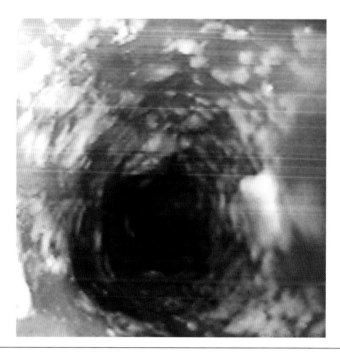

Figure 4.7 ● Severe *Candida* esophagitis.   The circumferential plaque material coats at least 50% of the esophageal mucosa.

of the mucosa. With disease progression, the plaques themselves can narrow the esophageal lumen (Fig. 4.7) (5).

   Ulceration from *Candida* esophagitis is very rare. When ulceration is seen, consideration for concomitant viral etiologies should be made, most commonly cytomegalovirus (5). Under the plaque, the mucosa is inflamed but without true ulceration. The infection generally remains limited to the superficial epithelium as a result of repeated shedding of the epithelium into the esophageal lumen. Histopathologic diagnosis is made by identification of yeast and mycelial forms typical for *Candida*. Treatment consists of topical antifungal agents such as nystatin and systemic antifungal agents such as fluconazole.

HERPES ESOPHAGITIS

Esophagitis due to herpes is the most frequent viral etiology of esophagitis. While herpes esophagitis typically presents in immunocompromised hosts, it also occurs in immunocompetent individuals. Squamous epithelium is the primary target of the herpes virus, so in the gastrointestinal tract, the esophagus is preferentially affected. Approximately 20% of patients with herpes esophagitis have concomitant oropharyngeal lesions (6). The most common presenting symptom is acute onset of severe odynophagia and dysphagia, with inability to handle secretions. The dysphagia resulting from herpes esophagitis can resemble dysphagia from acute cerebrovascular disease with the inability to handle secretions and drooling and can be severe enough to warrant nonoral means of nutritional support. Endoscopy reveals multiple, shallow ulcerations with raised, heaped-up edges, sometimes forming a large series of ulcers (7,8). The distal one third of the esophagus is most commonly affected. Biopsy of the edge of the ulcer assists in making the diagnosis, though tissue viral culture sometimes is necessary. Herpes esophagitis can be treated with acyclovir, though it can resolve spontaneously.

CYTOMEGALOVIRUS ESOPHAGITIS

Cytomegalovirus (CMV) esophagitis is the second most common viral cause of esophagitis and is typically seen in immunocompromised hosts. CMV involves the esophagus less frequently than herpes, as it does not infect squamous epithelial cells. Instead, it infects fibroblasts within granulation tissue and epithelium of submucosal glands. Therefore, the glandular mucosa of the stomach is more frequently affected with CMV than the esophagus. Patients with CMV esophagitis generally present with symptoms of odynophagia, with dysphagia as a rare presenting symptom. While there are no classic endoscopic characteristics of CMV esophagitis, the most common endoscopic features are esophageal ulceration and granulation tissue in contrast to the erosions usually seen with *Candida*. The esophageal ulcers are generally discrete lesions of varying depths with intervening normal mucosa. The ulcers are usually larger than 1 cm in diameter, and in about one third of cases, the ulcers are very large, i.e., greater than 2 cm (9). Most of the ulcers are located in the middle and distal esophagus. Diagnosis is made by biopsy of the ulcers (the rim and the central portion) and is confirmed by in situ DNA hybridization (10). Treatment options include intravenous ganciclovir and foscarnet and highly active antiretroviral therapy (11).

PILL-INDUCED ESOPHAGITIS

When an immunocompetent patient presents with relatively recent onset of odynophagia, acute retrosternal pain, and a history of taking a new medication, consideration must be given to pill-induced esophagitis. Pill-induced esophagitis is caused by prolonged contact of the esophageal mucosa with medication, resulting in inflammation and ulceration of the epithelium. This may occur in patients with normal esophageal motility (12). The etiology of esophageal injury is primarily due to one or more of several mechanisms (13):

(a) Direct caustic effect—clindamycin, potassium chloride, alendronate sodium, and quinidine
(b) Alteration of esophageal pH—tetracycline, clindamycin, ascorbic acid, and ferrous sulfate, causing an acid burn; phenytoin causing an alkali burn
(c) Accumulation of toxic levels of drugs within esophagus—doxycycline, nonsteroidal anti-inflammatory drugs
(d) Induction of reflux—anticholinergics, theophylline

Three antibiotics—doxycycline, tetracycline, and clindamycin—are responsible for over 50% of published cases of pill-induced esophageal injury (14). However, the most severe damage is caused by ascorbic acid, quinidine, potassium chloride, and alendronate sodium.

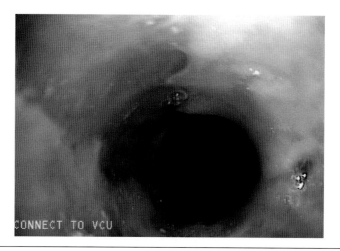

Figure 4.8 ● Pill-induced esophagitis with ulceration. Note the well-demarcated ulcer with surrounding area of grossly normal esophageal mucosa.

Endoscopy will reveal one or more well-demarcated ulcers with surrounding areas of grossly normal mucosa (Fig. 4.8) (15). Occasionally no ulceration is present, but what appears is diffuse inflammation with or without the presence of a pill remnant. While any portion of the esophagus may be injured, the most common site of injury is at the portion of the esophagus that passes posterior to the arch of the aorta (16). The treatment for pill-induced esophagitis involves taking pills with plenty of water, avoiding double swallowing, to be upright when taking the pills, to crush pills or take them in liquid form, and to not take them immediately before bedtime. In addition, empiric antacid therapy has become a mainstay of treatment.

CAUSTIC ESOPHAGITIS

Caustic injuries to the esophagus are more common in the pediatric population, generally the result of accidental ingestion. Caustic injuries in adults are usually the result of suicide attempts. Alkali injury, such as lye ingestion, is the most common cause of caustic injury to the esophagus (17). The extent of esophageal injury depends on the concentration of the ingested agent, the length of time tissue is exposed to the offending agent, and the status of the host (18). Stricture and stenosis as a result of caustic ingestion can occur along the entire upper aerodigestive tract, including the nasopharynx (Fig. 4.9) and hypopharynx (Fig. 4.10).

The endoscopic appearance of the esophagus as a result of caustic ingestion has been classified into three degrees, depending on the extent of the burn of the tissues:

- First-degree or superficial burns result in nonulcerative esophagitis or mild mucosal erythema and edema.
- Second-degree burns are transmucosal with shallow to deep ulceration and with possible extension to the muscularis. White exudates and severe erythema may also be seen.
- Third-degree burns show deep ulceration with possible perforation. Also, dusky, blackened transmural tissue with little remaining mucosa and possible obliteration of the esophageal lumen are seen with deep third-degree burns (19).

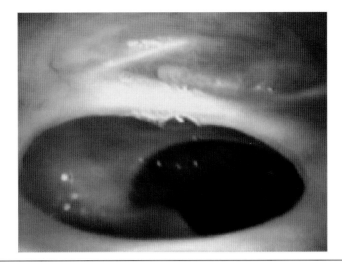

Figure 4.9 ● Lye injury to nasopharynx, causing nasopharyngeal stenosis. An oval band of scar tissue is at the level of the nasopharynx; the larynx is seen in the distance.

Alkali injuries are generally much more severe than acid injuries; as the alkali causes a liquefaction necrosis of tissue, there is no protective eschar and tissue penetration is extensive (20). In contradistinction, acid injury causes a coagulation necrosis whose depth is limited by eschar formation (21).

The immediate management of caustic injury involves volume support and control of infection. In addition, endoscopy is essential in evaluating the initial extent of injury and will guide subsequent management. The concern that esophagoscopy itself can potentially cause more injury is real (19); however, with smaller caliber instrumentation, such as that made

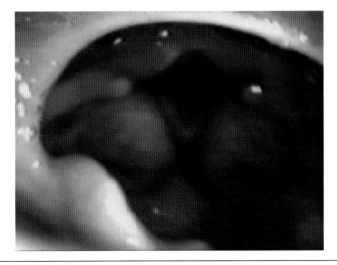

Figure 4.10 ● Lye injury to hypopharynx, causing hypopharyngeal stenosis. An oval band of scar tissue encompasses the epiglottis anteriorly.

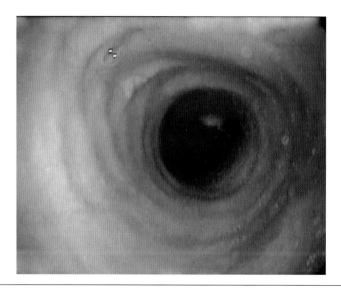

Figure 4.11 ● Eosinophilic esophagitis in an adult. Note the "trachealized" esophagus.

available by TNE, routine endoscopic surveillance of the esophagus can be readily performed. The late sequelae of caustic injury, in addition to dysphagia secondary to stricture and stenosis, includes esophageal motility problems and acid reflux disease (22). As a result, the long-term management of caustic injury to the esophagus should incorporate attention to dietary, behavioral, and medical management of reflux.

EOSINOPHILIC ESOPHAGITIS

Eosinophilic esophagitis (EE) is an uncommon inflammatory disorder with a possible allergic component, most commonly seen in children but now emerging as a disorder in adults as well. Adults usually present with chronic dysphagia for solids, food impaction, proximal strictures, or refractory gastroesophageal reflux symptoms.

Endoscopic findings include single or multiple "rings" or corrugations (so-called trachealization of the esophagus), small-caliber esophagus, proximal esophageal stenosis, and small whitish vesicles or exudate resembling *Candida*. (Fig. 4.11)

Biopsies demonstrating >15 eosinophils per HPF are diagnostic of EE. Treatment is orally administered fluticasone propionate twice daily for 6 weeks (23,24).

REFERENCES

1. Armstrong D, Bennett JR, Blum AL, et al. The endoscopic assessment of esophagitis: a progress report on observer agreement. *Gastroenterology* 1996;111:85–92.

2. Lundell LR, Dent J, Bennett JR, et al. Endoscopic assessment of esophagitis: clinical and functional correlates and further validation of the Los Angeles classification. *Gut* 1999;45:172–180.

3. Geisinger KR, Teot LA. Role of histology and cytology in esophageal disease. In: Castell DO, Richter JE, eds. *The esophagus*. 3rd ed. Philadelphia: Lippincott Williams & Williams; 1999:145–147.

4. Baehr PH, McDonald GB. Esophageal infections: risk factors, presentation, diagnosis and treatment. *Gastroenterology* 1994;106:509–532.

5. Wilcox CM, Schwartz DA. Endoscopic-pathologic correlates of Candida esophagitis in acquired immune deficiency syndrome. *Dig Dis Sci* 1996;41:1337–1345.

6. Ramanathan J, Rammouni M, Baran J Jr, et al. Herpes simplex virus esophagitis in the immunocompetent host: an overview. *Am J Gastroenterol* 2000;95:2171–2176.

7. Monkemuller KE, Wilcox CM. Diagnosis of esophageal ulcers in acquired immunodeficiency syndrome. *Semin Gastrointest Dis* 1999;10:85–92.

8. Amaro R, Poniecka AW, Goldeberg RI. Herpes esophagitis. *Gastrointest Endosc* 2000;51:68.

9. Wilcox CM, Straub RF, Schwartz DA. Prospective endoscopic characterization of cytomegalovirus esophagitis in AIDS. *Gastrointest Endosc* 1994:40:481–484.

10. Schwartz DA, Wilcox CM. Atypical cytomegalovirus inclusions in gastrointestinal biopsy specimens from patients with the acquired immunodeficiency syndrome: diagnostic role of in situ nucleic acid hybridization. *Hum Pathol* 1992;23:1019–1026.

11. Drew WL. Cytomegalovirus disease in the highly active antiretroviral therapy era. *Curr Infect Dis Rep* 2003;5:257–265.

12. Kikendall JW. Pill-induced esophageal injury. *Gastroentrol Clin North Am* 1991;20:835–846.

13. Chami TN, Nikoomanesh P, Katz PO. An unusual presentation of pill-induced esophagitis. *Gastrointest Endosc* 1995;45:263–265.

14. Jaspersen D. Drug-induced oesophageal disorders: pathogenesis, incidence, prevention and management. *Drug Saf* 2000;22:237–249.

15. Misra SP, Dwivedi M. Pill-induced esophagitis. *Gastrointest Endosc* 2002;55:81.

16. Kikendall JW. Pill esophagitis. *J Clin Gastroenterol* 1999;28:298–305.

17. de Jong AL, Macdonald R, Ein S, et al. Corrosive esophagitis in children: a 30-year review. *Int J Pediatr Otorhinolaryngol* 2001;57:203–211.

18. Kirsch MM, Ritter F. Caustic ingestion and subsequent damage to the oropharyngeal and digestive passages. *Ann Thoracic Surg* 1976;21:74–82.

19. Spiegel JR, Sataloff RT. Caustic injuries of the esophagus. In: Castell DO, Richter JE, eds. *The esophagus*. 3rd ed. Philadelphia: Lippincott Williams & Williams; 1999:561.

20. Friedman EM. Caustic ingestions and foreign bodies in the aerodigestive tract of children. *Pediatr Clin North Am* 1989;36:1403–1410.

21. Ein SH, Shandling B, Stephens CA. Twenty-one year experience with the pediatric gastric tube. *J Pediatr Surg* 1987;22:77–81.

22. Bautista A, Varela R, Villanueva A, et al. Motor function of the esophagus after caustic burn. *Eur J Pediatr Surg* 1996;6:204–207.

23. Noel RJ, Putnam PE, Collins MH, et al. Clinical and immunopathologic effects of swallowed fluticasone for eosinophilic esophagitis. *Clin Gastroenterol Hepatol* 2004;2:568–575.

24. Potter JW, Saelan K, Staff D, et al. Eosinophilic esophagitis in adults: an emerging problem with unique esophageal features. *Gastrointest Endosc* 2004;53:355–361.

5

Webs and Rings

The majority of esophageal webs and rings are found incidentally during esophagoscopy and are of no clinical significance. In certain individuals, however, they can be an important cause of dysphagia, and the endoscopist performing transnasal esophagoscopy (TNE) must be thoroughly familiar with their diagnosis and management.

RINGS

Lower esophageal rings are classified into two primary types. The A-ring is a thick, muscular ring found approximately 2 cm above the squamocolumnar junction. It marks the upper border of the lower esophageal sphincter (Fig. 5.1). Muscular A-rings are exceedingly rare. Although many clinicians consider them a variant of normal esophageal anatomy, they have been reported to cause dysphagia (1–3). Because the constriction caused by A-rings is secondary to muscular hypertrophy and not stricture formation, dilation is seldom successful at relieving the dysphagia. Botulinum toxin type A injections into the muscular ring have been shown to be beneficial but may result in a significant increase in reflux (3). Whereas the A-ring is muscular, the B-ring is a thin, annular membranous ring of mucosa associated with submucosal fibrosis at the gastroesophageal junction.

The B-ring is the classic Schatzki's ring. Schatzki's rings are the most common cause of solid food dysphagia in adults. They are seen in up to 14% of routine barium swallow examinations (1,2). The majority of esophageal rings are found incidentally and are of little significance. Although the exact etiology of Schatzki's rings is uncertain, it may be related to chronic gastroesophageal reflux disease. They are usually found at the squamocolumnar junction and are almost always associated with a hiatal hernia (Fig. 5.2). Squamous esophageal mucosa is seen on the proximal and gastric columnar mucosa on the distal surface of the ring. Gastroesophageal reflux disease should be considered in all patients, and ambulatory pH monitoring or empiric antireflux therapy should be performed in select patients (4,5). Schatzki's rings, when measured radiographically, tend to be symptomatic if the opening is <13 mm. Those that leave an 18- to 20-mm lumen are nearly always asymptomatic. Dilation of the B-ring is successful in relieving the dysphagia. This may be accomplished by mechanical dilation (bougienage) or disruption by pneumatic balloons using endoscopy or fluoroscopy. Care should always be taken when evaluating a patient using transnasal esophagoscopy because the smaller caliber endoscope may allow the examiner to miss esophageal rings, as well as mild strictures. In addition, the power of the air insufflator is less than the standard gastroenterology esophagoscope, and this limits our ability to distend the esophagus and visualize some rings and webs.

WEBS

In comparison to rings and strictures, esophageal webs are seen much less frequently. Like the Schatzki's ring, webs are mucosal in nature. They may occur anywhere along the length of the esophagus. Unlike the Schatzki's ring, which occurs at the esophageal-gastric junction, they must have squamous mucosa on both surfaces. Proximal webs have been primarily described in women with iron deficiency anemia with the eponyms Paterson-Kelly and Plummer-Vinson syndromes. It is usually seen in the cervical esophagus near the postcricoid region (Figs. 5.3 and 5.4). Webs in the postcricoid region can be missed on contrast studies, and therefore

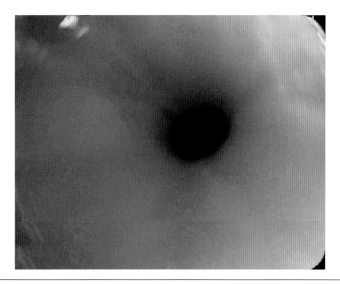

Figure 5.1 ● **Muscular A-ring seen above the squamocolumnar junction.**

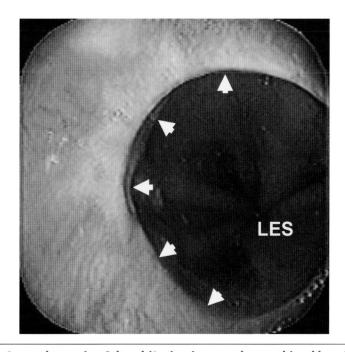

Figure 5.2 ● **A nonobstructive Schatzki's ring is seen above a hiatal hernia.** The lower esophageal sphincter (LES) is seen distal to this. Note the linear terminal vessels.

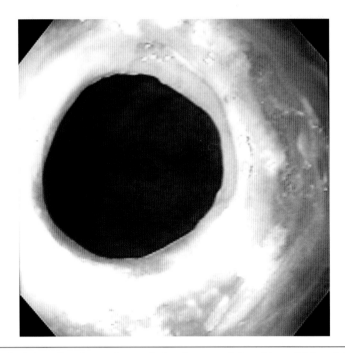

Figure 5.3 ● A tight, distal esophageal ring in an adult with solid food dysphagia.

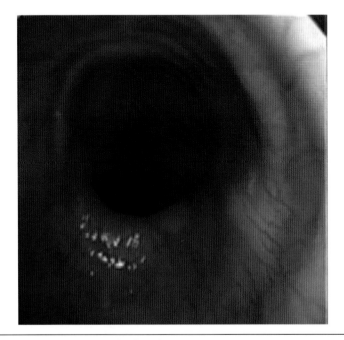

Figure 5.4 ● A symptomatic cervical web.

this area must be examined carefully in people with dysphagia. Routine dilation is usually curative.

REFERENCES

1. DeVault, Kenneth R. Lower esophageal (Schatzki's) ring: pathogenesis, diagnosis and therapy. *Dig Dis* 1996;14:323–329.

2. Jalil S, Castell DO. Schatzki's ring: a benign cause of dysphagia in adults. *J Clin Gastroenterol* 2002;35(4):295–298.

3. Wu W. Esophageal rings and webs. In: Castell DO, Richter JE, eds. *The esophagus.* 2nd ed. Boston: Little, Brown; 1995:337–343.

4. Hirano I, Gilliam J, Goyal RK. Clinical and manometric features of the lower esophageal muscular ring. *Am J Gastroenterol* 2000;95(1):43–49.

5. Varadarajulu S, Noone T. Asymptomatic lower esophageal muscular ring: response to Botox. *Dig Dis Sci* 2003;48:2132–2134.

6

Hiatal Hernia

Hiatal hernias (HH) are frequently encountered during routine transnasal esophagoscopy (TNE). The prevalence of hiatal hernia increases with age. Although the existence of a HH does not itself indicate the presence of gastroesophageal reflux disease, persons with a HH are prone to more severe reflux. The two mechanisms in which HH promotes reflux are through (a) a mechanically defective lower esophageal high-pressure zone and (b) the creation of a reservoir that allows for the expeditious regurgitation of gastric contents into the esophagus. Table 6.1 lists the means by which a HH contributes to a defective distal antireflux barrier. A thorough understanding of the anatomy of the distal antireflux barrier is necessary in order to accurately identify pathology in this region and to diagnose HH (1–3).

There are three primary contributors to the distal antireflux barrier. In order of decreasing importance they are: the intrinsic lower esophageal sphincter (LES), the diaphragmatic hiatus, and the valve effect created by the angle of His. The intrinsic LES is a 3- to 4-cm high-pressure zone at the gastroesophageal junction (GEJ). Although the endoscopist is unable to accurately differentiate the exact boundaries of the LES from the more proximal esophagus, the sphincter is a distinct entity that is tonically contracted at rest. The midpoint of the LES is at the approximate level of the squamocolumnar junction (SCJ). The normal anatomic relationship is such that the LES lies within the hiatus of the right diaphragmatic crura. The phrenoesophageal ligaments serve to anchor the LES at about the level of the SCJ (Fig. 6.1). These distinctions can be blurred when the gastric mucosa migrates into the more proximal esophagus, such as with Barrett's esophagus, and when the LES migrates higher into the chest, as with HH. The diaphragmatic hiatus augments internal LES tone (4). When the hiatus is not at the level of the LES (HH), the resting LES tone is significantly lower (5). The key to evaluating the endoscopic presence of a HH is in being able to differentiate the GEJ from the crura of the diaphragm. The third contributor to the lower esophageal high-pressure zone is the valve effect created by the oblique entrance of the esophagus into the stomach at the angle of His (Fig. 6.1) (6).

The endoscopic evaluation of the GEJ is the most difficult part of esophagoscopy interpretation. The terms squamocolumnar junction and gastroesophageal junction are not synonymous. The term GEJ is reserved to describe the actual muscular or anatomic junction between the esophagus and stomach. The best way to endoscopically define the GEJ is to visualize the termination of the linear esophageal mucosal blood vessels from above meeting the gastric rugae from below (Fig. 6.2). The SCJ refers specifically to the junction between the squamous epithelium of the esophagus and the columnar epithelium of the stomach. In the

---

TABLE 6.1
Means by which hiatal hernia contributes to a defective antireflux barrier

- Rupture or stretching of phrenoesophageal ligament
- Loss of flap-valve effect of angle of His that bolsters the lower esophageal sphincter (LES)
- Loss of intra-abdominal LES (negative pressure of chest cavity reduces LES pressure)
- Loss of support from diaphragmatic hiatus
- Shortening of LES

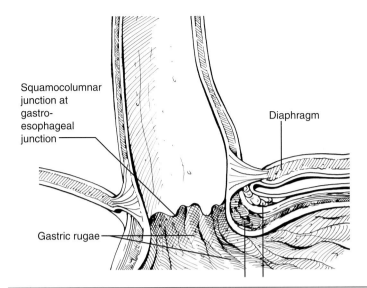

Squamocolumnar junction at gastro-esophageal junction

Diaphragm

Gastric rugae

Figure 6.1 ● The lower esophageal antireflux barrier.   Note that the squamocolumnar junction and gastroesophageal junction are at the same location and on the same plane as the diaphragm.

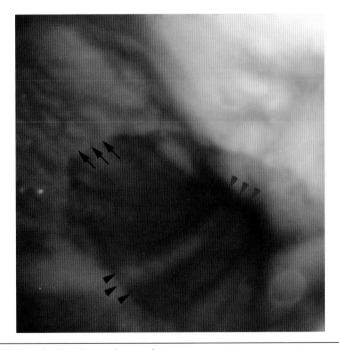

Figure 6.2 ● Normal distal esophageal anatomy.   The squamocolumnar junction (SCJ) is at the level of the gastroesophageal junction (GEJ). The SCJ marks the transition between esophageal squamous and gastric columnar epithelium (*black arrows*). The GEJ is identified by the termination of the linear esophageal mucosal vessels (*black arrows*) and the most proximal extent of the gastric rugae (*black arrowheads*). The GEJ is 1.5 cm above the diaphragmatic hiatus (*blue arrowheads*). A type I hiatal hernia exists when the GEJ is ≥2 cm above the hiatus.

normal esophagus (i.e., no Barrett's metaplasia), the SCJ is at the level of the GEJ, both of which are at the level of the diaphragmatic hiatus or pinch. The location of the hiatus can be confirmed with the patient performing the "sniff" maneuver that causes a "pinching" or rapid reduction in the diameter of the esophageal lumen. With insufflation of air distending the esophagus, the gastric folds may normally extend up to 2 cm above the hiatus. Proximal migration of the rugae 2 cm or more above the hiatus indicates the presence of a HH (Fig. 6.3). Judging length during TNE is based on the diameter of the transnasal endoscope (~0.5 cm). The circumference of the SCJ is usually irregular or serrated. The proximal border of the LES is best visualized endoscopically just superior to the rosette of linear esophageal mucosal folds (Fig. 6.4).

The most common type of HH is a sliding, or type I HH (Fig. 6.5A). A type I HH exists when the GEJ migrates out of the abdominal cavity into the posterior mediastinum of the chest. There are two primary ways to diagnose a type I HH endoscopically. The first is to visualize the gastric folds 2 cm or more above the hiatus (Fig. 6.6). The second is to visualize a defect in the hiatus with migration of the gastric rugae into the mediastinum on the retroflexed view (Fig. 6.7).

A type II or paraesophageal HH exists when the GEJ is anchored in the peritoneal cavity but a large defect in the hiatus allows a portion of the stomach to migrate into the mediastinum. Paraesophageal hiatal hernias represent less than 5% of all hernias (Fig. 6.5B). A type

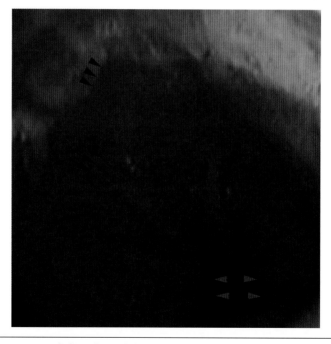

Figure 6.3 ● A type I sliding hiatal hernia (HH).   The proximal extent of the gastric folds marks the gastroesophageal junction (GEJ) (*black arrows*). The GEJ is 3.5 cm above the diaphragmatic hiatus (*blue arrowheads*). This defines the presence of a type I HH. Note that the squamocolumnar junction (*black arrowheads*) is 2 cm above the GEJ. This suggests the presence of short (<3 cm) Barrett's metaplasia. Biopsy of this region is necessary to confirm the diagnosis.

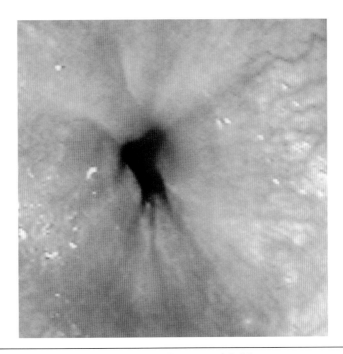

Figure 6.4 ● Rosette of linear esophageal mucosal folds. This represents an approximation of the proximal border of the intrinsic lower esophageal sphincter.

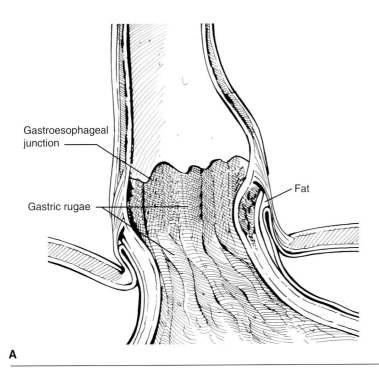

Gastroesophageal junction

Gastric rugae

Fat

A

Figure 6.5 ● Types of hiatal hernia (HH). **A.** A type I sliding HH. Note the gastroesophageal junction (GEJ) and squamocolumnar junction are well above the diaphragmatic hiatus.

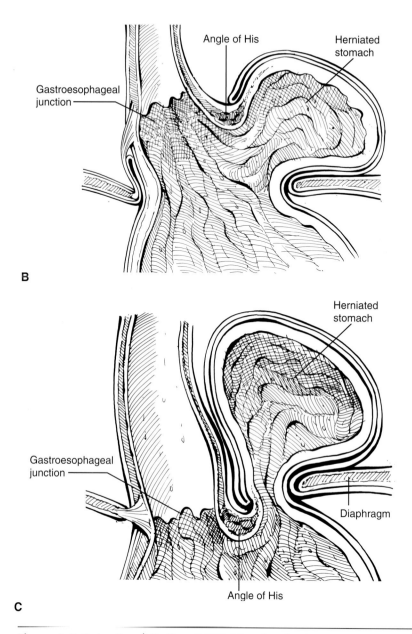

Figure 6.5 ● *(continued)* **B.** Type II HH. Note that the GEJ remains at the level of the diaphragm. **C.** Type III HH. Note the loss of the angle of His.

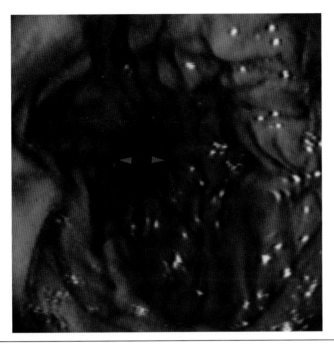

Figure 6.6 ● Endoscopic view within a large type I hiatal hernia sac. The rugae extend 5 cm above the hiatus (*blue arrowheads*). The squamocolumnar junction and gastroesophageal junction are proximal to this view and are not visualized on this image.

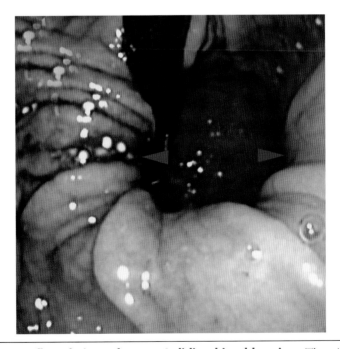

Figure 6.7 ● Retroflexed view of a type I sliding hiatal hernia. There is a 1.5-cm defect in the hiatus (*blue arrowheads*) with proximal migration of the gastric folds into the chest. The size of the defect is estimated by using the diameter of the esophagus (0.5 cm) as a guide.

III or mixed HH exists when both the GEJ and a portion of the gastric body or fundus migrate into the chest (Fig. 6.5C). Type II and III HHs can be difficult to diagnose endoscopically. They are best evaluated with retroflexion, where the extension of the hernia sac into the chest can be differentiated from the GEJ around the endoscope.

REFERENCES

1. Fein M, Ritter MP, DeMeester TR, et al. Role of the lower esophageal sphincter and hiatal hernia in the pathogenesis of gastroesophageal reflux disease. *J Gastrointest Surg* 1999;3:405–410.

2. Gordon C, Kang JY, Neild PJ, et al. The role of the hiatus hernia in gastro-oesophageal reflux disease. *Aliment Pharmacol Ther* 2004;20:719–732.

3. Orlando RC. Overview of the mechanisms of gastroesophageal reflux. *Am J Med* 2001; 111(Suppl 8A):174S–177S.

4. Klein WA, Parkman HP, Dempsey DT, et al. Sphincterlike thoracoabdominal high pressure zone after esophagogastrectomy. *Gastroenterology* 1993; 105: 1362 1369.

5. Kahrilis PJ, Lin S, Chen J, et al. The effect of hiatus hernia on gastro-esophageal junction pressure. *Gut* 1999;44:476–482.

6. Thor KB, Hill LD, Mercer DD, et al. Reappraisal of the flap valve mechanism in the gastroesophageal junction. A study of a new valvuloplasty procedure in cadavers. *Acta Chir Scand* 1987; 153(1):25–28.

7

Barrett's Metaplasia

INTRODUCTION

Barrett's esophagus (BE) is a replacement of the distal esophageal squamous mucosa with columnar-lined epithelium of both gastric and intestinal types (1). Today, Barrett's esophagus is defined as the presence of columnar appearing mucosa anywhere within the esophagus and specifically refers to intestinal metaplasia that contains Alcian blue-positive goblet cells (2). A histologic diagnosis of intestinal metaplasia is necessary to make the diagnosis of BE. When there are ≤3 cm of columnar epithelium protruding into the squamous epithelium of the esophagus, it is defined as short segment BE (Fig. 7.1) (3). When there are >3 cm of columnar epithelium extending into the esophagus, it is defined as long segment BE (Fig. 7.2). Because most instances of esophageal adenocarcinoma have BE as a precursor, it is necessary to be able to recognize the endoscopic features of BE. This requires a thorough understanding of distal esophageal endoscopic anatomy. (See Chapters 3 and 6.)

There are four items the endoscopist must recognize and evaluate in order to identify the presence of BE. These are the terminal linear esophageal blood vessels, the lower esophageal sphincter (LES), the squamocolumnar junction (SCJ), and the gastroesophageal junction (GEJ). The LES is generally located 38 to 41 cm from the nasal vestibule. When only a small amount of air is insufflated into the esophagus, the normotensive LES can typically be identified as a closed rosette of esophageal mucosal folds. The LES rests at the distal, coned-down end of several longitudinal, symmetrical esophageal mucosal folds (Fig. 7.3). Because this re-

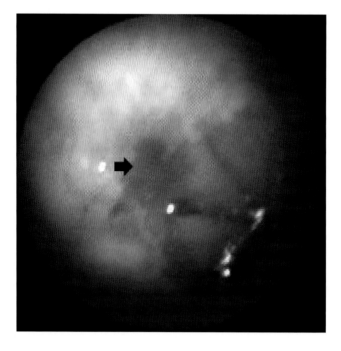

Figure 7.1 ● Short segment Barrett's esophagus (*black arrow*). Note the presence of a small lip of pink, mushroom-shaped epithelium at 10 o'clock, protruding into the esophageal squamous appearing mucosa along an irregular Z-line. This area of epithelium is extending <3 cm in length.

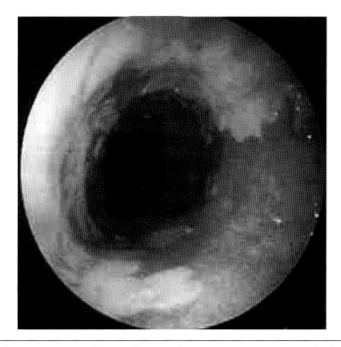

Figure 7.2 ● Long segment Barrett's esophagus.   A pink tongue of columnar-appearing epithelium >3 cm in length is extending into the esophagus.

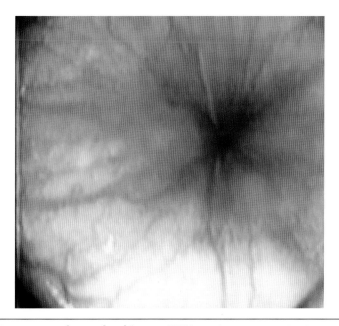

Figure 7.3 ● Lower esophageal sphincter (LES).   The LES is nearly closed and located at the distal portion of six longitudinal, symmetrical, esophageal mucosal folds. Where the LES is closed represents the location of the diaphragmatic pinch.

gion is where the diaphragmatic crura "pinches" the esophagus as it passes through the diaphragm, this area is also known as the "diaphragmatic pinch." The anatomic relationship of the LES and the diaphragm will be distorted in the presence of a hiatal hernia, and the gastric rugae will be above the diaphragmatic pinch.

The SCJ is normally at the level of the GEJ. The SCJ is the point where the gray-white squamous epithelium of the esophagus ends and the salmon- or pink-colored columnar epithelium of the stomach begins (Fig. 7.4). The SCJ usually appears as a slightly irregular demarcating line also known as the "Z-line." Several linear, gastric folds terminate at the level of the normal location of the squamocolumnar junction. The upper margin of these longitudinal gastric folds also corresponds to the level of the GEJ and provides a very useful landmark for the muscular junction between stomach and esophagus (Fig. 7.5). When the Z-line (SCJ) is located above the GEJ, there is columnar-lined epithelium in the esophagus.

The SCJ normally rests at, or just below, the level of the diaphragmatic pinch. When the proximal margins of the gastric folds, along with the normal squamocolumnar junction, are endoscopically present ≥2 cm above the diaphragmatic pinch, it is defined endoscopically as a hiatal hernia (Fig. 7.6) (4).

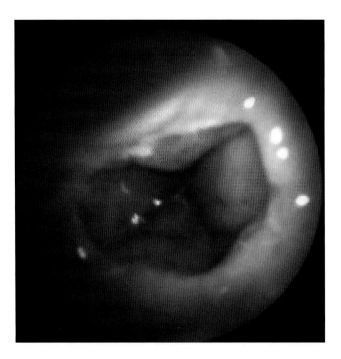

Figure 7.4 ● Normal squamocolumnar junction. This is the Z-line, which is the point where the gray-white squamous epithelium of the esophagus ends and the pink-colored columnar epithelium of the stomach begins.

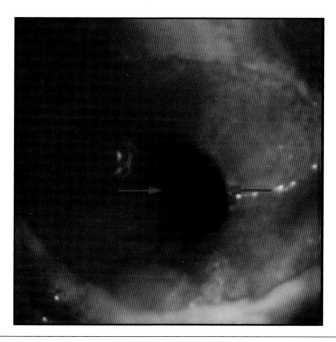

Figure 7.5 ● Normal gastroesophageal junction (GEJ). The GEJ is the point where the upper margin of the longitudinal gastric folds terminates at the level of the normal location of the squamocolumnar junction. The *blue arrows* point to the opening of the diaphragmatic hiatus.

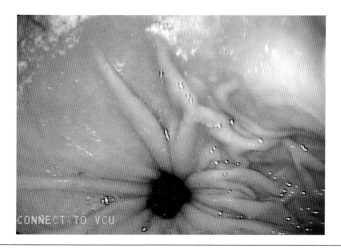

Figure 7.6 ● Hiatal hernia. Note the presence of gastric folds above the diaphragmatic pinch.

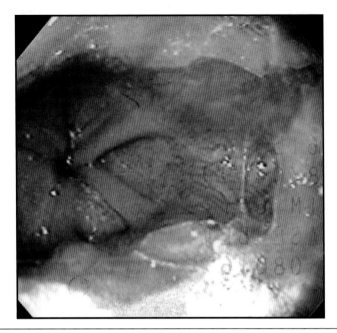

Figure 7.7 ● Barrett's esophagus with hiatal hernia. There is a large segment of pink epithelium at 2 o'clock, protruding into the gray-white squamous epithelium of the esophagus. Also, there are gastric rugae above the diaphragmatic pinch, signifying a hiatal hernia.

There are several endoscopic findings that suggest the presence of BE:

(a) The presence of a hiatal hernia. BE rarely occurs without a hiatal hernia (Fig. 7.7) (2).
(b) The squamocolumnar junction is proximal to the EGJ. In other words, the Z-line is orad to the gastric rugal folds, and the terminal linear vessels are covered by salmon-pink mucosa (Fig. 7.8).
(c) Tongues of columnar epithelium protruding into the esophageal squamous epithelium (Fig. 7.9).
(d) Islands of squamous epithelium below the squamocolumnar junction.

Barrett's esophagus is believed to be the precursor of dysplastic changes that can eventually progress to adenocarcinoma of the esophagus, which is the fastest rising malignancy in the United States over recent decades (3).

The incidence of esophageal adenocarcinoma in patients with BE is estimated to be 0.5% per year (5). It is thought to occur through a progression from Barrett's metaplasia to dysplasia to adenocarcinoma. Low-grade dysplasia has been shown to progress to cancer with an incidence of 12% over a 5-year period (6), while high-grade dysplasia progresses in up to 25% over the same period (7). Based on this information, the American College of Gastroenterology screening recommendations differ based on biopsy results, with surveillance for nondysplastic Barrett's metaplasia recommended every 3 years, low-grade dysplasia every year, and high-grade dysplasia every 3 months (or esophagectomy) (8). The importance of detecting dysplastic changes in biopsy specimens is well recognized but also fraught with challenges. Most

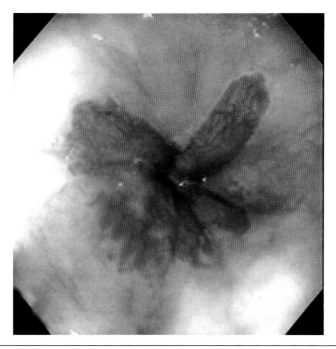

Figure 7.8 ● Squamocolumnar junction above diaphragmatic pinch.   Note that the Z-line is located above the GEJ, so by definition there exists columnar-lined epithelium in the esophagus.

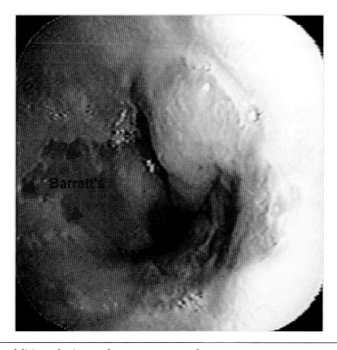

Figure 7.9 ● Additional view of Barrett's esophagus—tongue of columnar epithelium protruding into esophageal squamous epithelium.

individuals with symptomatic esophageal adenocarcinoma present with advanced disease with abysmal 5-year survival rates below 10%. If detected early via screening examinations, the survival rate can be improved to 80%. Provocative work by Reavis et al. suggests that screening of individuals with laryngopharyngeal reflux (LPR), particularly chronic cough, may result in improved detection of dysplasia and esophageal adenocarcinoma at earlier stages (9).

The prevalence of BE among patients with gastroesophageal reflux disease is estimated to range from 5% to 20% (10–13). Little is known about the prevalence of BE in LPR patients. One study with limited sample size (N = 58) found Barrett's metaplasia in 7% of LPR patients, but no further studies are available to corroborate this data (14).

REFERENCES

1. Barrett NR. Chronic peptic ulcer of the esophagus and "esophagitis." *Br J Surg* 1950; 38:175–182; Barrett NR. The lower esophagus lined by columnar epithelium. *Surgery* 1957; 41:881–894.

2. Boyce HW. Barrett esophagus: endoscopic findings and what to biopsy. *J Clin Gastroenterol* 2003;36(Suppl 5):S6–S18.

3. Spechler SJ. Barrett's esophagus. *N Engl J Med* 2002;346:836–842.

4. Boyce HW. Endoscopic definition of esophagogastric junction regional anatomy. *Gastrointest Endosc* 2000;51:586–592.

5. Coppola D, Karl RC. Barrett's esophagus and Barrett's associated neoplasia: etiology and pathologic features. *Cancer Control* 1999;6:21–27.

6. Reid BJ, Levine DS, Longton G, et al. Predictors of progression to cancer in Barrett's esophagus: Baseline histology and flow cytometry identify low- and high-risk patient subsets. *Am J Gastroenterol* 2000;95:1669–1676.

7. Cameron AJ, Carpenter HA. Barrett's esophagus, high-grade dysplasia, and early adenocarcinoma: a pathological study. *Am J Gastroenterol* 1997;92:586–591.

8. Sampliner RE. Updated guidelines for the diagnosis, surveillance, and therapy of Barrett's esophagus. *Am J Gastroenterol* 2002;97:1888–1895.

9. Reavis KM, Morris CD, Gopal DV, et al. Laryngopharyngeal reflux symptoms better predict the presence of esophageal adenocarcinoma than typical gastroesophageal reflux symptoms. *Ann Surg* 2004;239:849–856; discussion 856–858.

10. Toruner M, Soykan I, Ensari A, et al. Barrett's esophagus: prevalence and its relationship with dyspepsia symptoms. *J Gastroenterol Hepatol* 2004;19:535–540.

11. Chang JT, Katzka DA. Gastroesophageal reflux disease, Barrett esophagus, and esophageal adenocarcinoma. *Arch Inn Med* 2004;164:1482–1488.

12. Woolf GM, Riddell RH, Irvine EJ, et al. A study to examine the agreement between endoscopy and histology for the diagnosis of columnar-lined (Barrett's) esophagus. *Gastrointest Endosc* 1989;35:541–544.

13. Blot WJ, Devesa SS, Kneller RW, et al. Rising incidence of adenocarcinoma of the esophagus and gastric cardia. *JAMA* 1991;265:1287–1289.

14. Koufman JA, Belafsky PC, Bach KK, et al. Prevalence of esophagitis in patients with pH-documented laryngopharyngeal reflux. *Laryngoscope* 2002;112:1606–1609.

8

Neoplasia

INTRODUCTION

Most esophageal tumors are malignant. All esophageal lesions, benign or malignant, typically grow to a fairly large size before causing symptoms. The esophageal lumen usually needs to be significantly decreased (e.g., 20 mm down to 12–13 mm) before a patient complains of dysphagia. Therefore, patients typically present late in the course of their disease. Early detection of malignant or dysplastic lesions would likely result in improved survival. With the advent of unsedated transnasal esophagoscopy, there is a good likelihood that more frequent examination of the esophagus will result in the detection of esophageal neoplasms at an earlier stage. This may ultimately portend a better outcome for patients with esophageal cancer.

Cup biopsy forceps or biopsy brushes can be readily used to sample the vast majority of exophytic or flat intraluminal lesions. Care should be taken in the decision to biopsy submucosal or potentially vascular lesions due to the possibility of uncontrolled bleeding. The key to the evaluation of submucosal lesions is endosonography.

BENIGN ESOPHAGEAL NEOPLASMS

Most benign esophageal tumors, except for fibrovascular polyps, are located in the distal two thirds of the organ. Benign esophageal tumors can be classified clinically into those found within the lumen, whether mucosal or submucosal, and those that are extraluminal. Extraluminal esophageal neoplasms are more common than luminal tumors (1).

Leiomyoma

Leiomyomas are the most common benign esophageal neoplasm (2). They generally occur in men between the second to fifth decade of life. They are found in the distal esophagus, where smooth muscle predominates. The endoscopic appearance is a discrete bulging of the esophageal lumen without disruption of the mucosa. In addition, leiomyomas are mobile and the esophagoscope can be passed readily across the area of luminal narrowing. The diagnosis of leiomyoma is very difficult to make endoscopically and thus is generally made on radiographic examination of the esophagus or during endoscopic ultrasound (3).

Esophageal Cyst

Esophageal cysts are the second most common benign esophageal tumor and can be further classified into the more common inclusion cysts (intramural), or duplication cysts (extramural) (3,4). Esophageal cysts are typically asymptomatic and are found incidentally during radiographic examination of the esophagus or during endoscopy. The inclusion cysts are usually found in the upper esophagus adjacent to the tracheal bifurcation. They are generally managed without surgery. In contradistinction, duplication cysts primarily occur in the lower third of the esophagus, and their lining may consist of gastric mucosa, thereby producing acid. Acid-producing duplication cysts can cause ulceration; thus excision of these cysts are generally recommended (5). Because they are extraluminal, their endoscopic appearance is characterized by a vague narrowing of the esophageal lumen without disruption of the mucosa.

Fibrovascular Polyp

Fibrovascular polyps are the most common benign *intraluminal* tumor (6). Generally they are pedunculated, grow slowly, and can become quite long, some >20 cm (7,8). Because fibrovascular polyps grow and can cause obstruction or bleeding as necrosis of the tip of the polyp occurs, excision is recommended (9).

Granular Cell Tumor

Granular cell tumors are rare and typically asymptomatic. Over half are found in the distal one-third of the esophagus (3). Clinically they appear as smooth, oval, submucosal polypoid masses that are firm, pale, yellow, and sessile. They are generally <2 cm in diameter (10). Granular cell tumors are rarely malignant (1%–3%) and do not transform into malignancies (11,12).

Lipoma

Lipomas are rare submucosal tumors that are detected during esophagoscopy as a bulging of the overlying esophageal mucosa. Lipomas typically arise in the upper one third of the esophagus and are soft and pale yellow (Fig. 8.1). While lipomas generally do not require follow-up, there are cases where lipomas can grow to large sizes and cause obstructive symptoms (2,13).

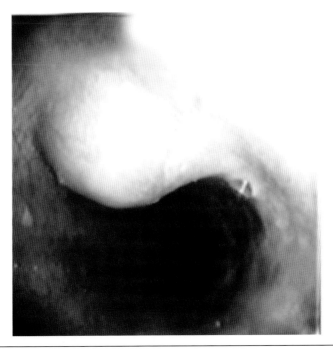

Figure 8.1 ● Lipoma. A soft, pale, yellow submucosal mass causes a bulging of the overlying esophageal mucosa.

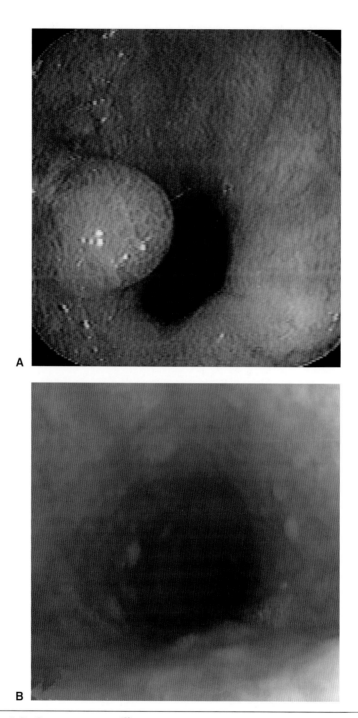

Figure 8.2 ● A,B. Squamous papilloma. Note the small, wart-like, sessile mass.

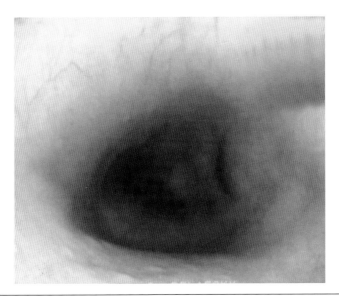

Figure 8.3 ● Hemangioma.   There is a mucosal-covered, discrete, raised lesion with a blue hue.

Papilloma

Squamous papillomas are rare, benign esophageal tumors. They are found incidentally during esophagoscopy as subcentimeter, sessile masses with a wart-like appearance (Fig. 8.2). Biopsy differentiates these benign lesions from superficial squamous cell carcinomas. Esophageal squamous papillomas rarely progress to malignancy (14).

Hemangiomas

Hemangiomas account for <3% of all benign esophageal tumors. On endoscopy, they appear as mucosal-covered, slightly raised, discrete, bluish-colored lesions that may be mistaken for varices (Fig. 8.3). Biopsy may result in extensive hemorrhage (15).

Inflammatory Pseudotumor

Inflammatory pseudotumors of the esophagus are uncommon benign lesions of the esophageal lumen. On endoscopy, they are usually pedunculated masses located in the distal third (Fig. 8.4). They can enlarge, cause mucosal ulceration, and appear malignant. Biopsy is necessary to confirm the diagnosis (16).

Lymphangioma

Lymphangiomas of the esophagus are exceedingly rare. On esophagoscopy, they appear as easily compressed, translucent, cystic masses. Biopsy is necessary to confirm the diagnosis. No follow-up is needed (17).

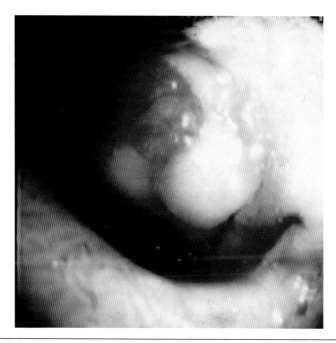

Figure 8.4 ● Inflammatory pseudotumor. Note the pedunculated mucosal-covered mass in the distal third of the esophagus.

MALIGNANT ESOPHAGEAL NEOPLASMS

Most esophageal neoplasms are malignant. Esophageal cancer had traditionally been thought of as a primarily squamous cell cancer. Adenocarcinoma of the esophagus, however, is the fastest growing cancer in the United States and is now more common than its squamous cell counterpart (18). Dysphagia is the most common presenting symptom of malignant esophageal tumors.

Squamous Cell Carcinoma

Squamous cell carcinomas of the esophagus appear most commonly in the middle third of the esophagus, followed in decreasing frequency by the distal third, and least commonly in the proximal third (1). Patients with head and neck cancer are at high risk for esophageal squamous cell cancers and should be screened with esophagoscopy (19). Patients with squamous cell cancer who are symptomatic will have some measure of luminal narrowing on esophagoscopy (Fig. 8.5A,B). In addition, the esophageal mucosa will often be friable and notable for an area of central ulceration with surrounding raised edges. The changes in the esophageal mucosa may appear more subtle, with color change or change in elevation of a segment of the tissue relative to the surrounding mucosa (20).

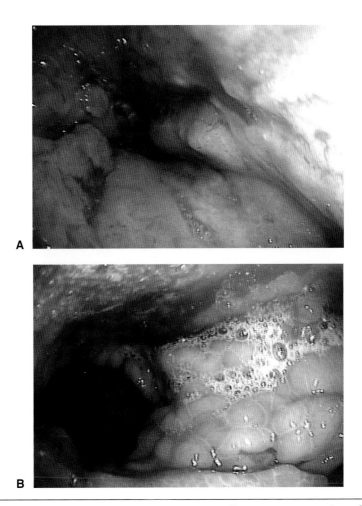

Figure 8.5 ● A. Advanced esophageal squamous cell carcinoma. B. Size of the tumor seen with retroflexion.

Adenocarcinoma

Adenocarcinoma of the esophagus has had a marked increase in incidence in the United States and Western Europe over the past three decades. It is most commonly seen in males and is almost always found in the distal third of the esophagus. Reports from the 1980s showed that patients with Barrett's esophagus (BE) have an incidence of adenocarcinoma from 40 to 125 times the incidence of the general population (18,21). The endoscopic findings in esophageal adenocarcinoma often show an area of BE adjacent to the area of the adenocarcinoma. The appearance of adenocarcinoma, in addition to the presence of an area of BE, can be a mucosal-covered nodule (Fig. 8.6). In more advanced cases, frank ulceration and esophageal narrowing can be observed (Figs. 8.7 and 8.8A,B).

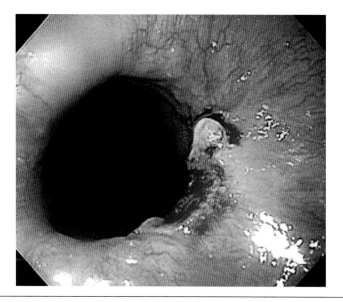

Figure 8.6 ● Early adenocarcinoma of esophagus. Note the subtle elevation of the esophageal mucosa relative to its surrounding tissue.

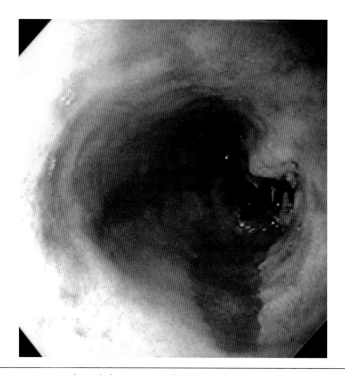

Figure 8.7 ● Barrett's and nodular mass of an esophageal adenocarcinoma. There is salmon-colored mucosa with raised nodules and without ulceration.

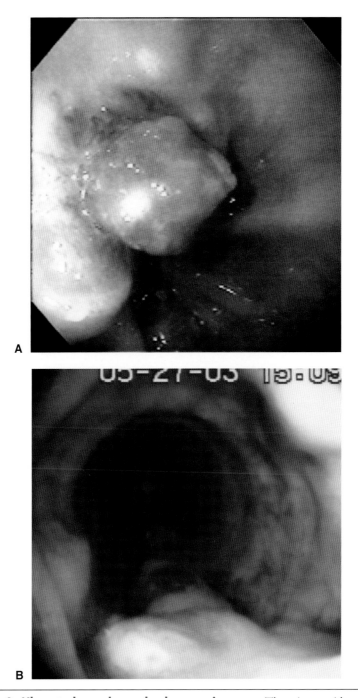

A

B

Figure 8.8 ● A. Ulcerated esophageal adenocarcinoma. There is no evidence of Barrett's epithelium; what is seen is frank ulceration and esophageal narrowing. Contrast with **(B),** showing submucosal spread of a squamous cell carcinoma.

REFERENCES

1. Fleischer DE, Haddad NG. Neoplasms of the esophagus. In: Castell DO, Richter JE, eds. *The esophagus.* 3rd ed. Philadelphia: Lippincott Williams & Williams; 1999:239–252.

2. Rice TW. Benign esophageal tumors: esophagoscopy and endoscopic esophageal ultrasound. *Semin Thorac Cardiovasc Surg* 2003;15:20–26.

3. Choong CK, Meyers BF. Benign esophageal tumors: introduction, incidence, classification, and clinical features. *Semin Thorac Cardiovasc Surg* 2003;15:3–8.

4. Overhaus M, Decker P, Zhou H, et al. The congenital duplication cyst: a rare differential diagnosis of retrosternal pain and dysphagia in a young patient. *Scand J Gastroenterol* 2003; 38:337–340.

5. Diaz de Liano A, Ciga MA, Trujillo R, et al. Congenital esophageal cysts: two cases in adult patients. *Hepatogastroenterology* 1999;46:2405–2408.

6. Schmied C, Roedel H, Bernardi M, et al. Fibrovascular polyp of the esophagus. *Gastrointest Endosc* 2002;55:80.

7. Lewis BS, Waye JD, Khilnani MT, et al. Fibrovascular polyp of the esophagus. *Mt Sinai J Med* 1988;55:324–325.

8. Belafsky P, Amedee R, Zimmerman J. Giant fibrovascular polyp of the esophagus. *South Med J* 1999;92:428–431.

9. Eliashar R, Saah D, Sichel JY, et al. Fibrovascular polyp of the esophagus. *Otolaryngol Head Neck Surg* 1998;118:734–735.

10. Brandimarte G, Tursi A, Vittori I, et al. Granular cell tumor of the oesophagus: a rare cause of dysphagia with differential diagnosis of oesophageal neoplastic lesions. *Dig Liver Dis* 2000; 32:803–806.

11. Norberto L, Urso E, Angriman I, et al. Yttrium-aluminum-garnet laser therapy of esophageal granular cell tumor. *Surg Endosc* 2002;16:361–362.

12. Kinney T, Waxman I. Treatment of benign esophageal tumors by endoscopic techniques. *Sem Thoracic Cardiovasc Surg* 2003;15:27–34.

13. Samad L, Ali M, Ramzi H, et al. Respiratory distress in a child caused by lipoma of the esophagus. *J Pediatr Surg* 1999;34:1537–1538.

14. Mosca S, Manes G, Monaco R, et al. Squamous papilloma of the esophagus: long-term follow up. *J Gastroenterol Hepatol* 2001;16:857–861.

15. Yoshikane H, Suzuki T, Yoshioka N, et al. Hemangioma of the esophagus: endosonographic imaging and endoscopic resection. *Endoscopy* 1995;27:267–269.

16. Saklani AP, Pramesh CS, Heroor AA, et al. Inflammatory pseudotumor of the esophagus. *Dis Esophagus* 2001;14:274–277.

17. Yoshida Y, Okamura T, Ezaki T, et al. Lymphangioma of the oesophagus: a case report and review of the literature. *Thorax* 1994;49:1267–1268.

18. Conio M, Blanchi S, Lapertosa G, et al. Long-term endoscopic surveillance of patients with Barrett's esophagus. Incidence of dysplasia and adenocarcinoma: a prospective study. *Am J Gastroenterol* 2003;98:1931–1939.

19. Murakami S, Hashimoto T, Noguchi T, et al. The utility of endoscopic screening for patients with esophageal or head and neck cancer. *Dis Esophagus* 1999;12:186–190.

20. Makary MA, Kiernan PD, Sheridan MJ, et al. Multimodality treatment for esophageal cancer: the role of surgery and neoadjuvant therapy. *Am J Surg* 2003;69:693–700.

21. Hameeteman W, Tytgat GN, Houthoff HJ, et al. Barrett's esophagus: development of dysplasia and adenocarcinoma. *Gastroenterology* 1989;96:1249–1256.

9

Miscellaneous Esophageal Disorders

Esophageal Diverticula

Esophageal diverticula are out-pouchings of the esophageal wall. They may contain all histo-logic sections of the wall or may lack the muscularis layer. These can be classified on the basis of their location or etiology. The most common classification is anatomical and divides esophageal diverticula into hypopharyngeal (Zenker's diverticulum), midesophageal diverticula, and epiphrenic diverticula.

Zenker's diverticula are a protrusion of the hypopharyngeal mucosa in the area of congenital weakness (Killians' dehiscence) between the inferior pharyngeal constrictor and the cricopharyngeus muscle. The presence of a diverticulum should always be suspected in patients with dysphagia and regurgitation or frequent coughing while eating. During transnasal esophagoscopy (TNE), if the examiner has difficulty intubating the esophagus, the patients very often will have either an undiagnosed Zenker's diverticulum or a hypertonic upper esophageal sphincter (1). During the initial part of the esophagoscopy, if the examiner sees food or copious secretions, then she/he should suspect that they are in a diverticulum, and great care should be taken not to cause a perforation of this "false lumen." Suctioning and judicious use of air insufflation coupled with a clockwise twisting of the esophagoscope should allow the esophageal lumen to come into view. The examiner should not aggressively advance the esophagoscope if the lumen is not visible to avoid perforation. Figure 9.1 demonstrates a Zenker's diverticulum during TNE.

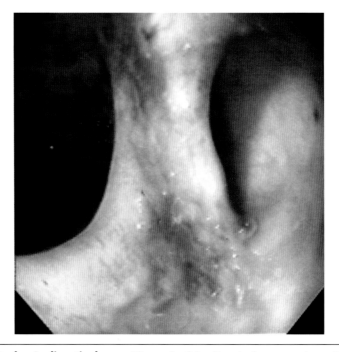

Figure 9.1 ● **Zenker's diverticulum.** The neck of the diverticulum opens into a large pouch. The esophageal lumen is to the patient's right.

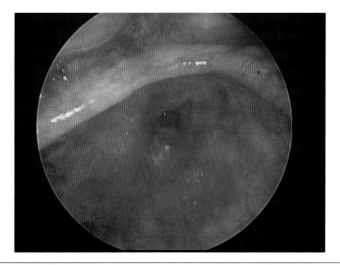

Figure 9.2 ● **Postsurgical scarring** adjacent to the lumen of the esophagus, allowing the diversion of some food into the pouch.

Dysphagia following the endoscopic treatment of these diverticula is uncommon but may result from scar formation across the site of the stapled diverticulotomy, as demonstrated in this patient 3 years after surgery (Fig 9.2).

The majority of midesophageal diverticula are asymptomatic due to the wide opening into their sacs. They generally represent old granulomatous disease that retracts the esophageal wall. They are usually diagnosed incidentally during a contrast esophagram (Fig. 9.3). Epiphrenic diverticula are often associated with esophageal motility disorders such as achalasia or diffuse esophageal spasm. Such diverticula can also develop proximal to esophageal strictures (Fig. 9.4).

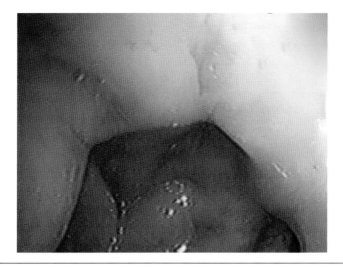

Figure 9.3 ● **An asymptomatic epiphrenic diverticulum** seen during esophageal screening in a patient with gastroesophageal and laryngopharyngeal reflux.

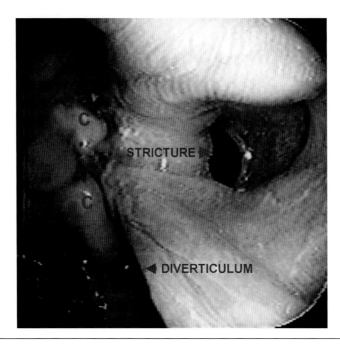

Figure 9.4 ● **A large diverticulum** seen proximal to a reflux induced stricture. Yesterday's lunch (corn) is seen. The patient underwent treatment with Savary dilators using transnasal esophagoscopy in the clinic, and his dysphagia resolved.

Esophageal Foreign Body

We do not advocate the removal of foreign bodies from the esophagus in the clinic using currently available technology. However, we use TNE to evaluate individuals who have a questionable history of foreign body ingestion and in patients whom we believe the foreign body is located in the distal esophagus and can be gently advanced into the stomach (2,3). Total or near-total obstruction may result in accumulated secretions and food that the examiner is unable to fully remove with the small-caliber suction channel. This may make evaluation and pushing the object into the stomach impossible.

The majority of adults having a foreign body impaction have a definite etiology for their difficulties. This is usually secondary to inflammation from gastroesophageal reflux, peptic or malignant stricture, esophageal dysmotility, neoplasm, or Schatzki's ring. It is important that the cause for the obstruction be established to enable appropriate therapy. Our technique involves gently suctioning any debris adjacent to the foreign body, and care is taken not to force the foreign body into a carcinoma or into an unappreciated esophageal diverticulum (Fig. 9.5). Air is insufflated to dilate the esophagus. The esophageal mucosa around the foreign body can then be evaluated. When the surgeon's clinical judgment is such that the foreign body can be advanced into the stomach, it is done with a combination of air insufflation, gentle pushing with the endoscope, and grasping with the biopsy forceps (Figs. 9.6 and 9.7). After the foreign body is advanced into the stomach, the entire area is reexamined to make a diagnosis and to evaluate the area for signs of trauma. If any difficulty occurs, the patient is taken to the operating room for rigid endoscopy. Metallic or sharp foreign bodies are taken to the OR for rigid endoscopy and are not managed with TNE.

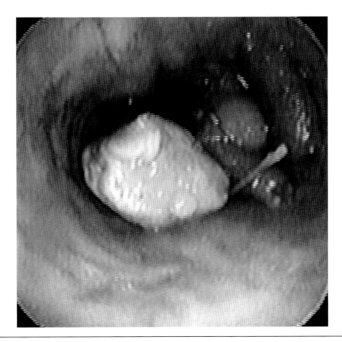

Figure 9.5 ● **Peppers seen proximal to a partially obstructing esophageal carcinoma.**

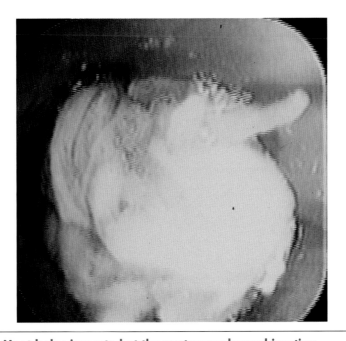

Figure 9.6 ● **Meat bolus impacted at the gastroesophageal junction.**

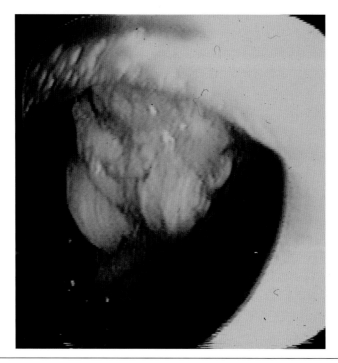

Figure 9.7 ● With air insufflation and gentle pressure, the foreign body is gently directed into the stomach.

Tracheoesophageal Fistula

Tracheoesophageal fistulas are fortunately uncommon entities. They are usually the consequence of a malignancy eroding the common wall between the trachea and esophagus. Less common etiologies would include chronic foreign bodies and trauma. Patients usually present with varying degrees of aspiration, dysphagia, chronic cough, frequent belching, or painful swallowing. The diagnosis is usually made via a barium swallow. Endoscopy can also provide the diagnosis. Small tears in the esophageal lumen can be missed unless a significant amount of air insufflation is provided to distend the esophagus. Bubbles may be seen in the secretions. Larger endoscopes can do this easily, while transnasal endoscopes are not as effective at significantly distending the esophagus with air. Figures 9.8 and 9.9 demonstrate a tracheoesophageal fistula from both the esophageal and tracheal view. This was a traumatic fistula which occurred during the dilation of this individual's tracheal stenosis and was not identified on barium swallow.

Esophageal Varices

Gastroesophageal variceal bleeding is a commonly encountered problem in patients with cirrhosis and portal hypertension. Varices are due to dilation of the collateral circulation between the portal vein and vena cava. Nearly all patients with cirrhosis will eventually develop esophageal varices. Fifty percent of cirrhotic patients will have endoscopic evidence of varices at the time of initial diagnosis. The risk of bleeding from these distended

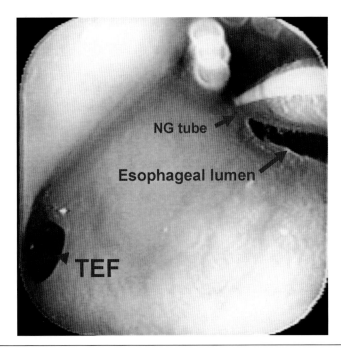

Figure 9.8 ● **The esophagoscope** is in the esophagus and the nasogastric tube and tracheo-esophageal fistula are seen.

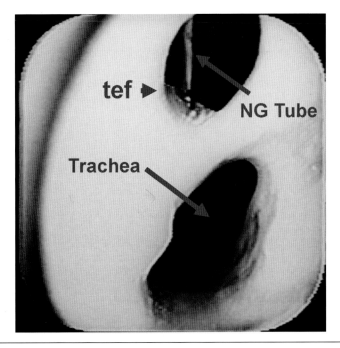

Figure 9.9 ● With the endoscope in the trachea, the tracheoesophageal fistula is well visualized.

submucosal veins is significant, and the overall mortality for a first variceal hemorrhage ranges from 17% to 57%. Many patients with esophageal varices will suffer from recurrent hemorrhage (4,5).

There remains controversy in the gastroenterologic literature regarding the proper care of patients with esophageal varices. Options include surveillance endoscopy, treatment with beta blockers, and preemptive treatment with various types of endoscopic therapy. In light of this, it is vital that the endoscopist be able to recognize these lesions and also avoid biopsying them during the course of a TNE. Esophageal varices appear as irregular, sometimes linear, sometimes tortuous submucosal lesions with a bluish hue. They may collapse with air insufflation. They can appear anywhere along the entire length of the esophagus, as well as in the gastric cardia, and as they enlarge, they can project into the lumen of the esophagus. Although varices do not typically break the mucosa, they can appear to be ulcerated if they have recently bled (Figs. 9.10 and 9.11). TNE may be the examination method of choice in cirrhotic patients and in patients following liver transplantation for variceal surveillance, since no sedation is needed in these often very ill and frail individuals. Care must be taken to not traumatize the nose, which could lead to difficult control of epistaxis in these patients.

Ultrathin endoscopy represents an advance in the diagnosis of esophageal disease, but the small operating channel does not allow therapeutic intervention for any type of bleeding. We recommend that submucosal lesions not be biopsied. These lesions should be evaluated with larger therapeutic endoscopes that can be used to control any significant bleeding during the specimen acquisition.

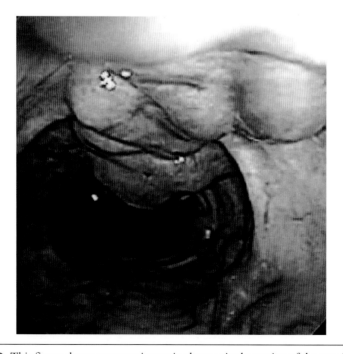

Figure 9.10 ● This figure shows an extensive varix along a single portion of the proximal esophagus.

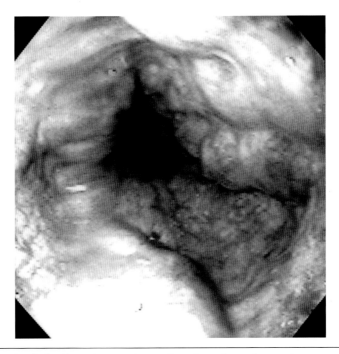

Figure 9.11 ● A cirrhotic with extensive varices throughout the esophagus encroaching on the esophageal lumen.

Anastomotic Evaluation

Transnasal esophagoscopy is a straightforward way to assess the suture line after hypopharyngeal and gastroesophageal surgery. The most common suture line that is assessed is the pharyngoesophageal segment after total laryngectomy (Fig. 9.12). In patients who have had a free-flap reconstruction or gastric pull-up after esophagectomy, TNE is a simple, easy way to evaluate the suture line and examine the region for recidivistic disease and strictures (Fig. 9.13) (6,7).

Achalasia

Achalasia is a failure of relaxation of the lower esophageal sphincter (LES). It is an esophageal disease of unknown etiology in which degeneration of neurons in the smooth muscle of the LES occurs so that the LES remains tonically contracted during a swallow. Over time, this can result in esophageal dilation and eventual loss of the contractile function of the esophageal body. During endoscopy, the LES will be difficult to traverse with the esophagoscope, and a pinhole opening may be all that is visualized in response to a swallow. Entry into the stomach is often difficult, and a palpable "pop" as the endoscopist enters the stomach has been described. The distal esophagus is often filled with secretions or food, is dilated, and may not demonstrate peristalsis. A retroflexed examination of the stomach and esophagus is needed to rule out a neoplastic obstruction mimicking achalasia, so-called secondary achalasia. The diagnosis is confirmed by barium swallow and manometry (Fig. 9.14). Treatment may involve dilation, injection of botulinum toxin type A into the LES, or myotomy.

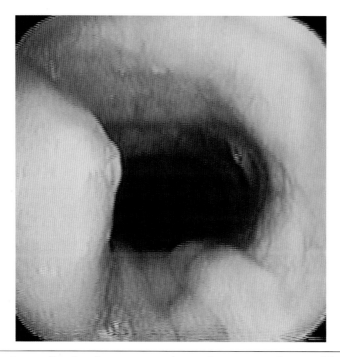

Figure 9.12 ● **Suture line in pharyngoesophageal segment after total laryngectomy.**

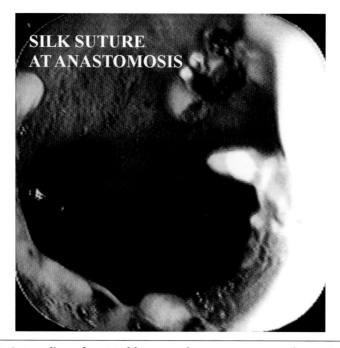

Figure 9.13 ● **Suture line after total laryngopharyngectomy and gastric pull-up.**

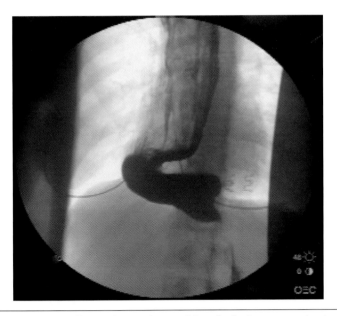

Figure 9.14 ● Barium swallow of a patient with achalasia. Note the classic "bird's beak."

Postfundoplication Evaluation

Complications after fundoplication occur in approximately 5% to 10% of individuals (8). In addition, recidivistic reflux symptoms may exist in up to 5% of individuals, and mild dysphagia may develop in up to 25% of individuals undergoing the procedure (9,10). Although we routinely obtain *both* barium esophagography and perform esophagoscopy in all persons requiring a postoperative fundoplication work-up, Jailwala et al. have shown that endoscopy is superior to esophagography in defining postsurgical abnormalities (11). A thorough knowledge of postoperative endoscopic findings is essential in order for the clinician to adequately evaluate and care for these individuals.

The goals of fundoplication are to reduce any existing hiatal hernia, restore the intraabdominal esophagus, reapproximate the diaphragmatic crura, and wrap the fundus around the esophagus to increase the distal esophageal high-pressure zone. The folds created by the wrapped fundus should be just below and parallel to the diaphragm, and the wrap should appear symmetric. When evaluating the integrity of a fundoplication, the endoscopist must first evaluate the distal esophageal mucosa to rule out esophagitis, dysplasia, carcinoma, and Barrett's esophagus (BE). The wrap zone may incorporate the distal esophagus and conceal the distal extent of a metaplastic segment or the entire region of a short segment BE. This can make postoperative fundoplication surveillance of BE and dysplasia more difficult. After evaluating the esophageal mucosa, the relationship between the gastroesophageal junction (GEJ) and the location of the wrap must then be assessed. The GEJ should be within 1 cm of the wrap. Any distance greater than 1 cm indicates a slipped fundoplication (stomach proximal to the fundoplication (Figs. 9.15 and 9.16). The endoscope must then be passed through the wrap into the stomach. The endoscopist notes the resistance to passage of the endoscope when traversing the wrap zone. An excessively tight or loose wrap is noted. Once the endoscope is in

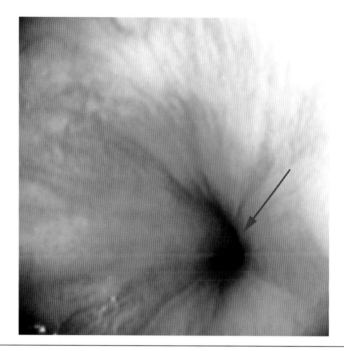

Figure 9.15 ● **Normal postfundoplication GEJ–fundoplication relationship.** The GEJ is at the level of the wrap (*blue arrow*).

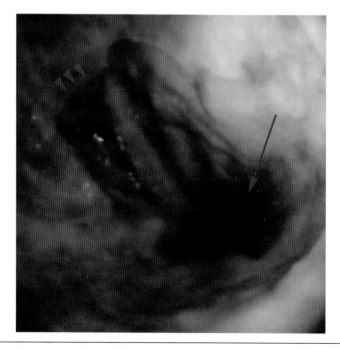

Figure 9.16 ● **Gastroesophageal junction** (*blue arrowheads*) 2 cm proximal to the wrap zone (*blue arrow*). This indicates a slipped fundoplication where the stomach has migrated above the wrap.

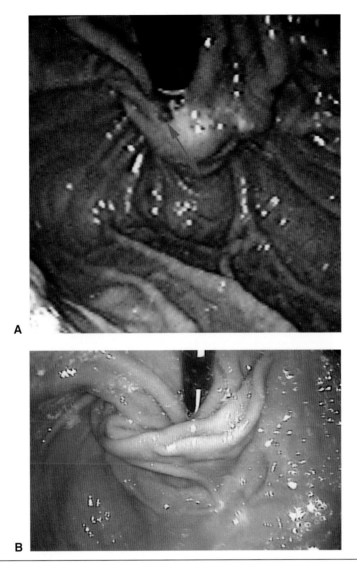

**Figure 9.17 ● A,B. Normal retroverted endoscopic images of an intact Nissen fundo-
plication.** The wrap can be seen as a cuff of rugal folds (*blue arrows*) parallel to the distance marking
on the endoscope. If the folds are not parallel, the fundoplication may be twisted.

the stomach, a retroflexed view of the GEJ is obtained, and the integrity of the fundoplication
is evaluated. An intact fundoplication has a very characteristic appearance on retroflexed view
(Fig. 9.17A,B). If this is not seen, the wrap may be disrupted or twisted (Fig. 9.18). If the wrap
is not snug around the endoscope, then the fundoplication is too patulous or incompetent.

Vascular Rings

Vascular rings caused by congenital anomalies of the aortic arch and its branches are an infre-
quent cause of dysphagia and airway compromise in adults. They are usually diagnosed in

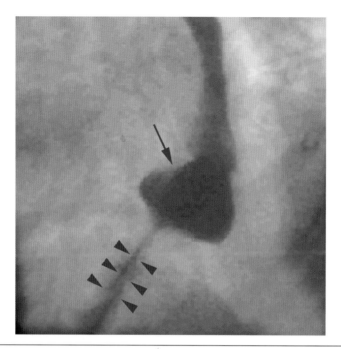

Figure 9.18 ● Barium esophagogram of a slipped fundoplication. The proximal stomach (*red arrow*) has herniated above the diaphragm and fundoplication. *Blue arrowheads* indicate the wrap-zone.

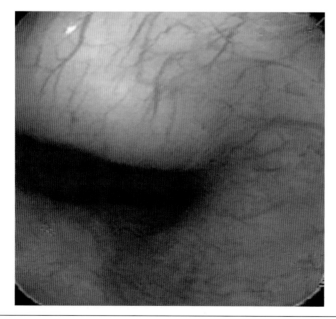

Figure 9.19 ● Dysphagia lusoria. Posterior compression of the esophagus by an aberrant right subclavian artery seen on transnasal esophagoscopy.

early infancy but may, at times, elude diagnosis until later in life. Vascular rings may be partial or complete. The most common congenital abnormality of the aorta is an aberrant right subclavian artery (RSCA). This forms an incomplete vascular ring. Although most persons with this are asymptomatic, dysphagia may occur from the retroesophageal passage of the RSCA between the esophagus and the spine (dysphagia lusoria) (Fig. 9.19).

Atherosclerosis and changes in thoracic compliance with aging may contribute to symptom progression in adults (12). The prevalence of aortic arch anomalies in adult cadavers is 0.01% (13). The most common cause of a complete ring is a double aortic arch (DAA, 46%), followed by a right-sided aortic arch (RAA, 30%) (14). Respiratory symptoms are more common in children, and dysphagia is the most common presenting complaint in adults (14).

The diagnosis of a vascular ring is established with any combination of barium esophagogram, plain chest radiography, echocardiography, coronary angiography, bronchoscopy, esophagoscopy, computed tomography, and magnetic resonance imaging (MRI) (12,15). With a DAA, two large indentions are seen on barium esophagography in posterior-anterior view. Esophagography in RAA displays a large right-sided and a small left-sided indention. Echocardiography is useful to exclude alternative cardiac anomalies and to define the anatomy of the vascular ring. Esophagoscopy and bronchoscopy may be performed to document the degree of luminal narrowing and exclude alternative pathology (Fig. 9.20). MRI displays excellent anatomic detail and has largely replaced the more invasive angiography as the diagnostic tool of choice (16,17). Operative intervention, either through a sternotomy or thoracotomy, is indicated for most symptomatic vascular rings. Patients with vascular rings caused by nonpatent elements may be a candidate for video-assisted thoracoscopic surgery (18,19).

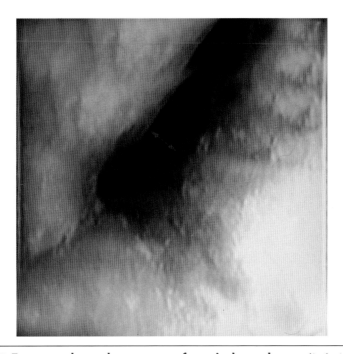

Figure 9.20 ● Transnasal esophagoscopy of cervical esophagus displaying compression from double aortic arch. Lumen is narrowed to 7 mm.

Esophageal Manifestations of Systemic Disease

There are numerous systemic diseases that can affect esophageal body and sphincteric function. The motility problems that ensue may predispose patients to symptoms of dysphagia, heartburn, cough, and regurgitation. Endoscopic findings that can occur as a consequence of the motility disorder include esophagitis, stricture, Barrett's metaplasia, and carcinoma.

Scleroderma

Scleroderma is a systemic connective tissue disease in which patients present with skin changes and Raynaud's phenomenon. The esophagus is affected in approximately 80% of cases (20). The disease causes fibrosis and atrophy of smooth muscle. Thus, the distal two thirds of the esophagus are affected and the proximal, striated muscle segment is spared. Barium esophagography and manometry reveal failed peristalsis along the distal two thirds of the esophagus and diminished LES pressures (21). Because of impaired esophageal motility and LES tonicity, patients with scleroderma will have symptoms and findings of severe acid reflux disease. In a normal swallow, the LES closes completely, and the endoscopic view of the LES is periodically obliterated as the result of a normal peristaltic wave. In patients with scleroderma, the squamocolumnar junction is visible throughout the swallow, and the normal obliteration of the esophageal lumen during a peristaltic wave does not take place. In addition, the LES does not close completely and may remain open throughout the swallow (Fig. 9.21). Mixed, connective tissue disease patients also manifest diminished esophageal motility, but the degree of dysfunction is usually not as severe as that seen in scleroderma (22).

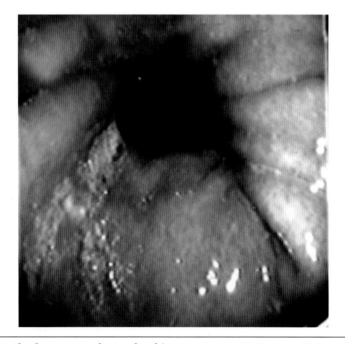

Figure 9.21 ● **The lower esophageal sphincter** remains widely patent before, during, and after swallow in a patient with scleroderma.

Epidermolysis Bullosa Dystrophica

Epidermolysis bullosa is a very uncommon disorder characterized by blister formation following minor skin trauma (23–26). In response to minor trauma such as that caused by food ingestion, there is disruption of the esophageal subepithelium with bullae formation. The functional esophageal findings include decreased peristalsis and esophageal atony. Additional endoscopic findings include strictures resembling webs, hiatal hernia, and pseudodiverticulum formation. Such individuals are usually placed on steroids for a few days prior to dilation.

Stevens-Johnson Syndrome

Stevens-Johnson syndrome is a rare, but severe, blistering mucocutaneous disease typically caused by an adverse reaction to medication (27). It can affect the esophagus and is characterized by complaints of dysphagia due to blistering and sloughing of the esophageal epithelium. Large ulcerations of the mucosa may occur along the entire length of the esophagus (Fig. 9.22) (28,29).

Glycogenic Acanthosis

Glycogenic acanthosis is a frequently seen incidental finding of unknown etiology and of no clinical significance. They appear as oval or round elevations usually <1 cm in size. Biopsy reveals enlarged hyperplastic epithelial cells with glycogen accumulation. It can occasionally be confused with small, flat esophageal papilloma. No follow-up is required (Fig. 9.23) (30).

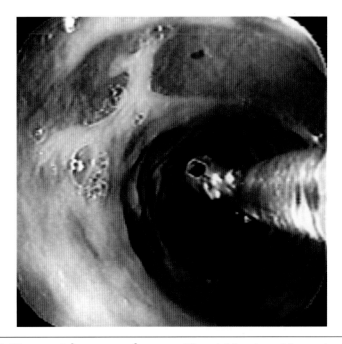

Figure 9.22 ● Stevens-Johnson syndrome. There is blistering of the esophageal mucosa with multiple ulcers.

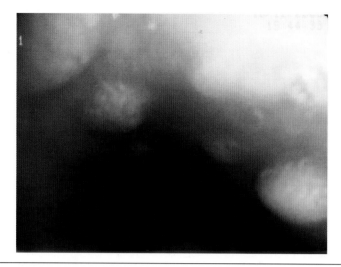

Figure 9.23 ● Classic appearance of glycogenic acanthosis in a patient with extra-esophageal reflux.

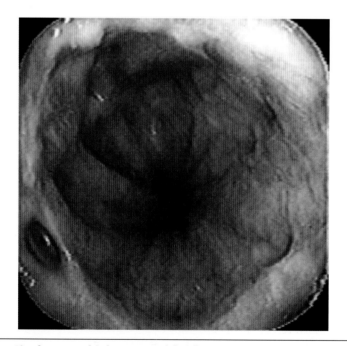

Figure 9.24 ● Single or multiple mucosal bridges are evidence of chronic gastroesophageal reflux disease. Antireflux therapy should hinder the cycle of inflammation and healing which is believed to produce them.

Mucosal Bridges

Mucosal bridging is occasionally seen in the distal esophagus and may be single or multiple. It is believed to be evidence of intermittent gastroesophageal reflux resulting in a cycle of inflammation and repair of the esophageal mucosa (Fig. 9.24).

REFERENCES

1. Postma GN, Belafsky PC. The evaluation of esophageal function with transnasal esophagoscopy. Presented at the American Academy of Otolaryngology Annual meeting, Orlando, FL, September 21, 2003.

2. Clyne S, Bach KK, Postma GN, et al. Foreign body in the esophagus. *Ear Nose Throat J* 2002;81:440.

3. Belafsky PB, Halsey WS, Postma GN, et al. Distal esophageal meat impaction. *Ear Nose Throat J* 2002;81:702.

4. Rigo GP, Merighi A, Chalen, NJ, et al. A perspective study of the ability of three endoscopic classifications to predict hemorrhage from esophageal varices. *Gastrointest Endosc* 1992; 38:425–429.

5. Graham D, Smith JL. The course of patients after variceal hemorrhage. *Gastroenterology* 1981;80:800–809.

6. Catalano MF, Sivak MV Jr, Rice TW, et al. Postoperative screening for anastomotic recurrence of esophageal carcinoma by endoscopic ultrasonography. *Gastrointest Endosc* 1995;42:540–544.

7. Lightdale CJ, Botet JF. Esophageal carcinoma: pre-operative staging and evaluation of anastomotic recurrence. *Gastrointest Endosc* 1990;36(2 Suppl):S11–S16.

8. Fuchs KH, Breithaupt W, Fein M, et al. Laparoscopic Nissen repair: indications, techniques and long-term benefits. *Langenbecks Arch Surg* 2005;390:197–202.

9. Catarci M, Gentileschi P, Papi C, et al. Evidence-based appraisal of antireflux fundoplication. *Ann Surg* 2004;239:325–337.

10. Beldi G, Glattli A. Long-term gastrointestinal symptoms after laparoscopic Nissen fundoplication. *Surg Laparosc Endosc Percutan Tech* 2002;12:316–319.

11. Jailwala J, Massey B, Staff D, et al. Post-fundoplication symptoms: the role for endoscopic assessment of fundoplication integrity. *Gastrointest Endosc* 2001;54:351–356.

12. Grathwohl KW, Afifi AY, Dillard TA, et al. Vascular rings of the thoracic aorta in adults. *Am Surg* 1999;65:1077–1083.

13. Bialowas J, Hreczecha J, Grzybiak M. Right-sided aortic arch. *Folia Morphol (Warsz)* 2000; 59:211–216.

14. Park MK. Vascular ring. In: Park MK. *Pediatric cardiology for practitioner*s. 4th ed. St. Louis: C.V. Mosby; 2002:241–246.

15. Greiner A, Perkmann R, Rieger M, et al. Vascular ring causing tracheal compression in an adult patient. *Ann Thorac Surg* 2003;75:1959–1960.

16. van Son JA, Julsrud PR, Hagler DJ, et al. Imaging strategies for vascular rings. *Ann Thorac Surg* 1994;57:604–610.

17. Azarow KS, Pearl RH, Hoffman MA, et al. Vascular ring: does magnetic resonance imaging replace angiography? *Ann Thorac Surg* 1992;53:882–885.

18. Burke RP. Video-assisted endoscopy for congenital heart repair. *Semin Thorac Cardiovasc Surg Pediatr Card Surg Annu* 2001;4:208–215.

19. Burke RP, Rosenfeld HM, Wernovsky G, et al. Video-assisted thoracoscopic vascular ring division in infants and children. *J Am Coll Cardiol* 1995;25:943–947.

20. Cameron AJ, Malcolm A, Prather CM, et al. Videoendoscopic diagnosis of esophageal motility disorders. *Gastrointest Endosc* 1999;49:62–69.

21. Spechler SJ, Castell DO. Classification of oesophageal motility abnormalities. *Gut* 2001; 49:145–151.

22. Weston S, Thumshirn M, Wiste J, et al. Clinical and upper gastrointestinal motility features in systemic sclerosis and related disorders. *Am J Gastroenterol* 1998;93:1085–1089.

23. Wong WL, Entwisle K, Pemberton J. Gastrointestinal manifestations in the Hallopeau-Siemens variant of recessive dystrophic epidermolysis bullosa. *Brit J Radiol* 1993;66:788–793.

24. Postma GN, Belafsky PC, Koufman JA. Dilation of an esophageal stricture caused by epidermolysis bullosa. *Ear Nose Throat J* 2002;81:86.

25. Travis SP, McGrath JA, Turnbull AJ, et al. Oral and gastrointestinal manifestations of epidermolysis bullosa. *Lancet* 1992;340:1505–1506.

26. Horan TA, Urschel JD, MacEachern NA, et al. Esophageal perforation in recessive dystrophic epidermolysis bullosa. *Ann Thoracic Surg* 1994;57:1027–1029.

27. Roujeau JC, Kelly JP, Naldi L, et al. Medication use and the risk of Stevens-Johnson syndrome or toxic epidermal necrolysis. *N Engl J Med* 1995;333:1600–1607.

28. Lamireau T, Leaute-Labreze C, Le Bail B, et al. Esophageal involvement in Stevens-Johnson syndrome. *Endoscopy* 2001;33:550–553.

29. Belafsky PC, Postma GN, Koufman JA, et al. Stevens-Johnson syndrome with diffuse esophageal involvement. *Ear Nose Throat J* 2002;81:220.

30. Vadva MD, Triadafilopoulos G. Glycogenic acanthosis of the esophagus and gastroesophageal reflux. *J Clin Gastroenterol* 1993;17:79–83.

10

Procedures

INTRODUCTION

Advances in technology over the past several years have enabled those interested in the aerodigestive tract to perform a wide array of procedures in the outpatient environment without sedation. Although techniques involving topical anesthesia have not changed appreciably, the extraordinary optical systems currently available with distal-chip transnasal esophagoscopes allow us to perform a variety of innovative procedures.

The success of office-based procedures is entirely dependent on the adequacy of the topical anesthesia and patient selection. Ideally, the patient selected for transnasal esophagoscopy (TNE) or any related procedures should not be overly anxious and should be confident that he or she can tolerate such a procedure. Virtually all our procedures are done through the nostrils, and therefore appropriate nasal patency is necessary. Anticoagulation is *not* a contraindication to TNE nor taking biopsies, but anticoagulated patients are observed for 15 minutes following the procedure to ensure that there is no bleeding.

Each procedure presented is performed with standard TNE anesthesia, as discussed earlier. In addition, 2 to 6 cc of lidocaine 2% to 4% is frequently administered through the working channel of the esophagoscope to the area of interest (pharynx, larynx, or trachea). This is usually all that is necessary for any procedure. No topical esophageal anesthesia is required for biopsies taken in the esophagus. Procedures in the trachea usually require additional topical anesthesia.

Other techniques for delivering topical anesthesia include dripping the anesthetic into the larynx and hypopharynx through a curved Abraham cannula passed transorally and the use of nebulized lidocaine. No matter which technique or anesthetic agent selected by the endoscopist, one must always keep in mind the recommended maximal dosages to avoid any adverse reactions to the local anesthetics. Lidocaine 4% has a maximal dose of 7 to 8 cc for a 70-kg patient (1).

Biopsies

The 2.0-mm working channel allows the passage of a 1.8-mm biopsy cup forceps. With adequate topical anesthesia, nearly any location in the upper aerodigestive tract can be biopsied without difficulty and without patient discomfort. We have biopsied lesions in the nasal cavity, nasopharynx, hypopharynx, larynx, subglottis, and trachea (Figs. 10.1 and 10.2). In addition, we routinely take biopsies throughout the esophagus and gastric cardia. We have obtained hundreds of biopsies without a single complication, and this includes biopsies taken from a number of individuals undergoing systemic anticoagulation with warfarin or clopidogrel bisulfate.

The use of the transnasal esophagoscope as a "panendoscope" for head and neck cancer patients provides the head and neck oncologic surgeon with a significant addition to his or her practice (2). This endoscope allows the biopsy of lesions, close detailed follow-up of head and neck cancer patients, as well as the avoidance of formal panendoscopy under general anesthesia in selected patients. An increasing number of our patients have undergone transnasal panendoscopy with biopsy, followed by definitive treatment without endoscopy and biopsy under general anesthesia (Fig. 10.3). Since TNE is so well tolerated without systemic medications, it is of great value in older individuals and in patients with significant medical comorbidities in whom sedation could be problematic.

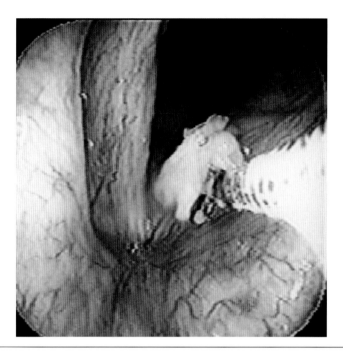

Figure 10.1 ● Biopsy of a left vocal-fold lesion using 1.8-mm cup forceps. The lesion was determined to be histoplasmosis.

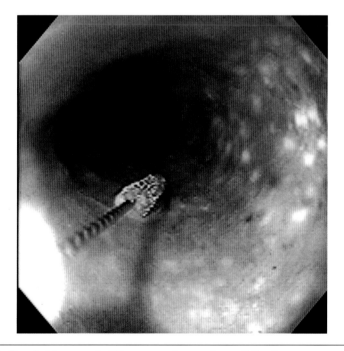

Figure 10.2 ● Brush biopsy of diffuse esophageal candidiasis.

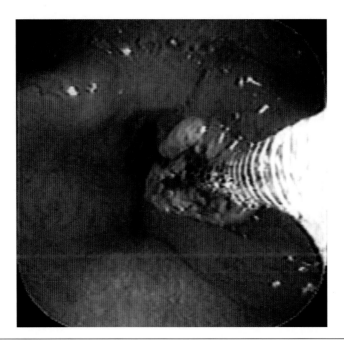

Figure 10.3 ● A diagnosis of supraglottic invasive squamous cell carcinoma is made.
Due to the small biopsy forceps, multiple biopsies are always taken.

Posttherapy Dysphagia

TNE can also assist in the evaluation of patients with dysphagia following cancer therapy and reconstruction. We occasionally feed patients with applesauce or water dyed with food coloring, or acetaminophen capsules while the esophagoscope is in place to evaluate the anastomotic sites of regional and free-flap reconstructions (Fig. 10.4) (3). This allows us to determine the precise location and cause of the individual's dysphagia.

Tracheoesophageal Puncture

Patients who have undergone total laryngectomy have many options for voice rehabilitation. In our practice, the most popular has been the placement of a voice prosthesis in a surgically created tracheoesophageal fistula. This can be performed in the office without sedation in properly selected patients (4). Such secondary tracheoesophageal punctures (TEP) can only be done in individuals with a reasonably sized tracheostoma. This procedure, when performed in the office, provides a significant cost saving. During the entire procedure, the transnasal esophagoscope provides the surgeon and assistant with clear visualization of the surgical site in the neopharynx by gentle insufflation of air. This allows the procedure to be done safely with a minimum of discomfort to the patient. In addition, the insufflation of air in the neopharynx in patients whose voice prosthesis has been lost allows reestablishment of the tracheoesophageal fistula and prosthesis reinsertion when it has partially closed (5).

In addition to the transnasal esophagoscope, a TEP dilator, as well as local anesthetic usually consisting of lidocaine 2% with epinephrine, and a No. 15 scalpel are employed. Patients

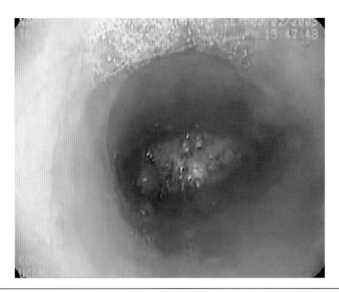

Figure 10.4 ● **Swallowing applesauce and/or acetaminophen capsules** can assist the surgeon in determining the site and cause of dysphagia.

undergoing this procedure should have neither neopharyngeal strictures nor a small stoma. Local anesthetic with epinephrine is infiltrated into the posterior tracheal wall at the area of the planned TEP site. After appropriate vasoconstriction has occurred, 2 cc of lidocaine 2% are sprayed into the tracheal stoma, the patient swallows 5 mL of a viscus lidocaine 2% solution, and the transnasal esophagoscope is then passed into the neopharynx. Both endoscopist and surgeon are now able to visualize the neopharynx. An 18- to 20-gauge needle is passed in the midline through the posterior tracheal wall, and the anterior wall of the esophagus is seen on the monitor (Fig. 10.5). The proper position is verified before penetration of the esophageal mucosa. Air insufflation protects the posterior esophageal wall. The needle is then withdrawn, and an incision is created in the same site using the scalpel blade (Fig. 10.6). A hemostat may be used to open this further if desired. The TEP dilators can then be passed under direct vision through the puncture site in the esophagus. We normally enlist the aid of one of our speech-language pathologists who uses the TEP sizing device, and then the appropriate size prosthesis is inserted. This is performed using the Gel-Cap technique. The Gel-Cap holds the inner flanges of the prosthesis together to allow it to be easily inserted. When it dissolves, the flange opens in the pharyngeal lumen. Positioning is verified using the endoscope. Alternatively, the placement of a red rubber catheter through the TEP is slightly easier than the immediate placement of a prosthesis (Fig. 10.7A,B). The catheter is secured to the neck with a 3-0 silk ligature. The fistula is allowed to mature for 72 hours, and the prosthesis is then placed by the speech language pathologist.

Pulsed-Dye Laser

The 585-nm pulsed-dye laser (PDL) has become increasingly popular in the management of laryngeal lesions, including recurrent respiratory papillomas (RRP), granulomas, and vocal-fold leukoplakia. The PDL energy penetrates epithelium without damaging it and is

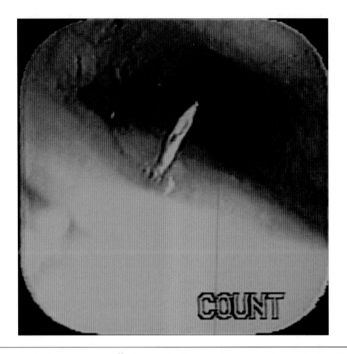

Figure 10.5 ● An 18-gauge needle is seen in the neopharyngeal lumen being distended open by air insufflation.

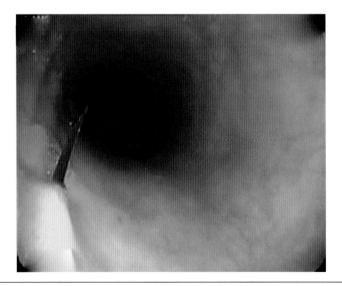

Figure 10.6 ● A scalpel opens the tracheoesophageal fistula.

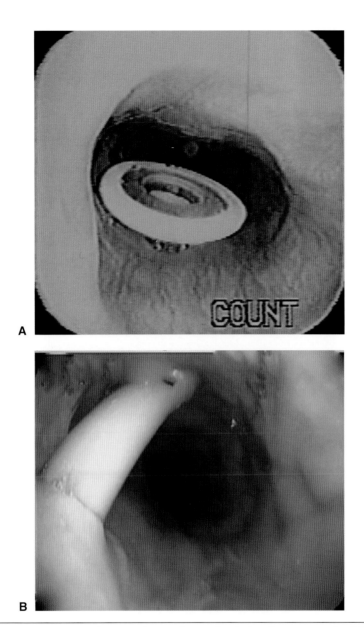

Figure 10.7 ● **A. The tracheoesophageal prosthesis in place. B. Red rubber catheter is shown.**

selectively absorbed by the underlying microvasculature (6–10). Because of its epithelium-sparing properties, otolaryngologists began to use the PDL for laryngeal lesions (11,12).

The indications are evolving but currently include RRP, chronic granulomas not responding to standard therapy (13), recurrent leukoplakia, Rienke's edema, and cancer palliation, and it may play a role in cancer therapy.

A flexible endoscope with a working channel or a sheath with a channel is required. We have employed a second endoscope through the other nostril which has been used for retraction of lesions in patients too ill for general anesthesia.

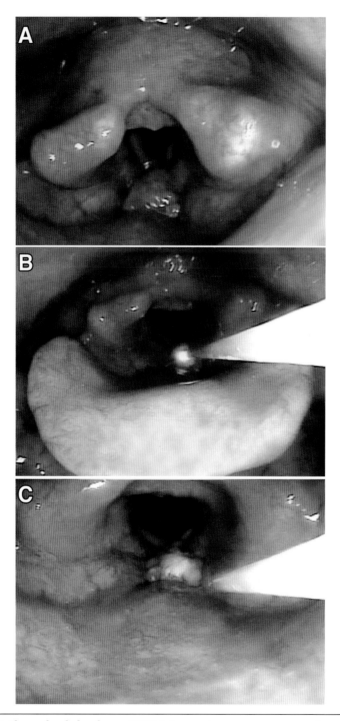

Figure 10.8 ● **The pulsed-dye laser (PDL)** being used to treat recurrent respiratory papillomas on the laryngeal surface of the epiglottis. **A.** The lesion that could not be exposed in the operating room via direct laryngoscopy is easily visualized in the clinic. **B.** The PDL fiber is millimeters from the surface of the lesion. **C.** The papilloma is blanched following treatment.

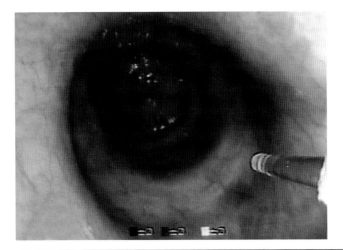

Figure 10.9 ● Ball-valving papilloma in the midtrachea.

The procedure is done in the office without sedation. Standard laser safety precautions are followed. These include laser equipment safety checklists and proper laser goggles for the patient and all individuals in the room. The patient is seated upright in an examination chair, and the more patent nostril is sprayed with 1:1 oxymetazoline 0.05% and lidocaine 4% and then packed with cotton pledgets using the same solution. The nasal packing is removed, and the TNE endoscope is lubricated and passed into the nasal cavity either along the floor of the nose or between the middle and inferior turbinates. When the larynx is in view, 4 to 8 cc of lidocaine 2% to 4% is sprayed onto the epiglottis and glottis through the working channel in the endoscope. The PDL fiber (PhotoGenica-SV; Cynosure Corporation, Chelmsford, MA) is passed through the port of the endoscope until the tip of the fiber is visible 1 to 2 cm past the tip of the endoscope. The tip of the fiber is then held close to the lesion (within several millimeters) and fired until the entire lesion blanches white (Fig. 10.8). The endoscope is then removed, and patients are allowed to go home from the clinic. Figures 10.9 to 10.11 show a large papilloma in the midtrachea being treated in this manner.

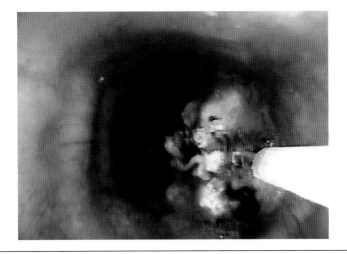

Figure 10.10 ● Extensive blanching is seen during the procedure.

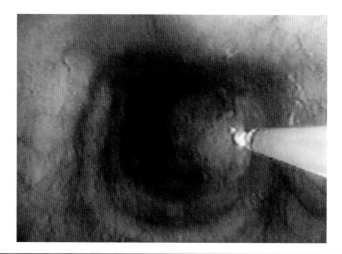

Figure 10.11 ● **One month following the initial treatment, the lesion has decreased markedly in size.**

Esophageal Dilation

Esophageal dilation can be performed in the clinic without sedation using a guidewire placed through the transnasal esophagoscope. This needs to be contrasted with the routine dilation of neopharyngeal strictures following laryngectomy performed "blindly" with Maloney dilators. This technique is used when direct visualization is needed, such as with a very narrow stricture, and a guidewire is passed. In addition to the transnasal esophagoscope, a set of Savary dilators with a vascular guidewire and a Kelly clamp is required. Savary dilators (Wilson-Cook Medical; Winston-Salem, NC) are progressively enlarging over-the-wire dilators (Fig. 10.12). Our technique begins with the insertion of the esophagoscope to directly visualize the stricture. The guidewire is then placed through the endoscope's working channel and advanced through the stricture under direct vision. The endoscope is then removed, and the guidewire is left in

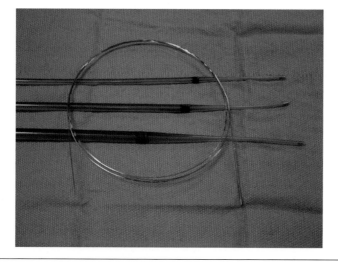

Figure 10.12 ● **Savary dilators with guidewire.**

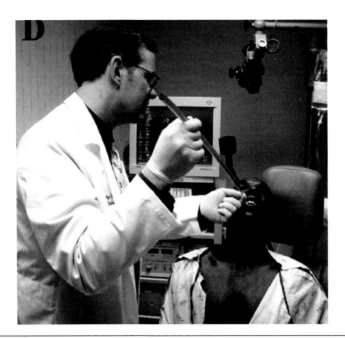

Figure 10.13 ● A Savary dilator is advanced over the guidewire.

place. At this time it is going from the patient's nose and passing through the area of stricture. The wire is then extracted with the Kelly clamp from the patient's mouth, and then the well-lubricated Savary dilators are placed over the wire and the stricture is gently dilated using sequentially larger dilators (Fig. 10.13) (14). Using an oral appliance for the esophagoscopy would allow the endoscopist to perform over-the-wire dilations without having to retrieve the guidewire from the nose. Another method involves passage of a hydrostatic balloon dilator transnasally alongside the endoscope and dilating the stricture under direct vision (Fig. 10.14).

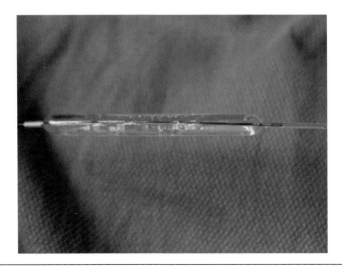

Figure 10.14 ● Hydrostatic balloon catheter.

Patients with severe strictures, such as high cervical strictures following radiation and chemotherapy, can be successfully treated using this technique coupled with sedation. Dr. Larry Johnson has treated a large number of such patients using Savary and even biliary dilators on a weekly treatment schedule with good results. In addition, Dr. Johnson describes using the TNE endoscope to assist in the placement of manometry catheters through the LES in patients with achalasia and a tortuous esophagus (15).

Placement of pH Probes

Ambulatory pH testing is an important element in the diagnosis and treatment of reflux disease. Ambulatory pH testing can be performed with a hard-wired pH probe or with a wireless pH telemetry capsule. The primary advantage of the hard-wired probe is the ability to place two or even three pH sensors at different locations throughout the upper aerodigestive tract. The primary disadvantage of the hard-wired test is the need for a transnasal catheter that is unsightly, uncomfortable, and reduces reflux-provoking behavior (16).

Ambulatory pH probes are typically placed by previously determined manometric parameters. The distal sensor is placed 5 cm above the upper border of the manometrically determined, lower esophageal high-pressure zone. Appropriate placement of a hypopharyngeal sensor is 1 cm above the proximal border of the upper esophageal sphincter (UES) (17,18). Alternatively, transnasal esophagoscopy can be utilized to localize the upper and lower esophageal sphincters and to determine the accurate position for pH probe placement (19). Once the locations of the sphincters are identified, either hard-wired or wireless pH sensors

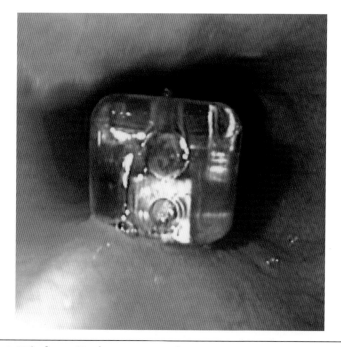

Figure 10.15 ● **Wireless pH telemetry capsule** secured 6 cm above the squamocolumnar junction.

may be placed. Correct endoscopic placement of a distal esophageal pH sensor is 6 cm above the squamocolumnar junction (SCJ). This has been shown to correspond to 5 cm above the proximal border of the lower esophageal high-pressure zone. When placing wireless pH probes, we prefer to pass the Bravo delivery catheter (Medtronic; Minneapolis, MN) immediately after TNE through the same dilated, anesthetized nare in which the endoscopy was performed. The capsule is placed 6 cm above the endoscopic determination of the SCJ. TNE may be repeated to confirm successful capsule placement (Fig. 10.15). Previous work has shown that an extraesophageal pH wire probe can be accurately placed 1 cm above the UES by direct endoscopic visualization in the majority of patients (20).

REFERENCES

1. Simpson CB, Amin MR, Postma GN. Topical anesthesia of the airway and esophagus. *Ear Nose Throat J* 2004;83(7 Suppl 2):2–5.

2. Postma GN, Bach KK, Belafsky PC, et al. The role of transnasal esophagoscopy in head and neck oncology. *Laryngoscope* 2002;112:2242–2243.

3. Bach KK, Postma GN, Koufman JA. Evaluation of flaps following pharyngoesophageal reconstruction. *Ear Nose Throat J* 2002;81:766.

4. Bach KK, Postma GN, Koufman JA. In-office tracheoesophageal puncture using transnasal esophagoscopy. *Laryngoscope* 2003;113:173–176.

5. Belafsky PC, Postma GN, Koufman JA. Replacement of a failed tracheoesophageal puncture (TEP) under direct vision. *Ear Nose Throat J* 2001;80:862.

6. Greenwald J, Rosen S, Anderson RR, et al. Comparative histological studies of the tunable dye (at 577nm) laser and argon laser: the specific vascular effects of the dye laser. *J Invest Dermatol* 1981;77:305–310.

7. Anderson RR, Parrish JA. Selective photothermolysis: precise microsurgery by selective absorption of pulsed radiation. *Science* 1983;220:524–527.

8. Tan OT, Kerschmann R, Parrish JA. The effect of epidermal pigmentation on selective vascular effects of pulsed laser. *Lasers Surg Med*. 1984;4:365–374.

9. Anderson RR, Parrish JA. Microvasculature can be selectively damaged during dye lasers: a basic theory and experimental evidence in human skin. *Lasers Surg Med* 1981;1:263–276.

10. Anderson RR, Jaenicke KF, Parrish JA. Mechanisms of selective vascular changes caused by dye lasers. *Lasers Surg Med* 1983;3:211–215.

11. Franco RA Jr, Zeitels SM, Farinelli WA, et al. 585-nm pulsed dye laser treatment of glottal papillomatosis. *Ann Otol Rhinol Laryngol* 2002;111:486–492.

12. Franco RA Jr, Zeitels SM, Farinelli WA, et al. 585-nm pulsed dye laser treatment of glottal dysplasia. *Ann Otol Rhinol Laryngol* 2003;112:751–758.

13. Clyne S, Halum S, Koufman JA, et al. Pulsed-dye laser treatment of laryngeal granulomas. *Ann Otol Rhinol Laryngol* 2005;114:198–201.

14. Postma GN, Belafsky PC, Koufman JA. Dilation of an esophageal stricture caused by epidermolysis bullosa. *Ear Nose Throat J* 2002;81:86.

15. L.F. Johnson, personal communication, 2004.

16. Fass R, Hell R, Sampliner RE, et al. Effect of ambulatory 24-hour esophageal pH monitoring on reflux-provoking activities. *Dig Dis Sci* 1999;44:2263–2269.

17. Postma GN, Belafsky PC, Aviv JE, et al. Laryngopharyngeal reflux testing. *Ear Nose Throat J* 2002;81(9 Suppl 2):14–18.

18. Kahrilas PJ, Lin S, Chen J, et al. The effect of hiatus hernia on gastro-oesophageal junction pressure. *Gut* 1999;44:476–482.

19. Belafsky PC, Allen K, Castro-Del Rosario L, et al. Wireless pH testing as an adjunct to unsedated transnasal esophagoscopy: the safety and efficacy of transnasal telemetry capsule placement. *Otolaryngol Head Neck Surg* 2004;131:26–28.

20. Johnson PE, Koufman JA, Nowak LJ, et al. Ambulatory 24-hour double-probe pH monitoring: the importance of manometry. *Laryngoscope* 2001;111(11 Pt 1):1970–1975.

INDEX

Page numbers in italics denote figures; those followed by a t denote tables.

ACG. *See* American College of Gastroenterology
Achalasia, 77, *79*
Acid injury, caustic esophagitis caused by, 33
Acid reflux
    as esophagitis etiology, 26, *27, 28, 29*
    HH and, 44, 44*t*
    pH testing and, 100
    scleroderma and disease of, 84
Acyclovir, herpes esophagitis treatment with, 31
Adenocarcinoma, 65
    appearance of, 65, *66*
    ulcerated, 65, *67*
Alendronate sodium, pill-induced esophagitis caused
        by, 31
Alkali injury, caustic esophagitis caused by, 32, 33
American College of Gastroenterology (ACG), 2
American Society for Gastrointestinal Endoscopy
        (ASGE), 2
Anastomotic evaluation, 77
Anesthesia
    hypopharynx, 13
    nasal cavity, 11, 13
    PDL, 97
    TNE and topical, 6, *6*
    nasal, 11
    techniques for delivering, 90
Anticoagulation, 90
Antireflux barrier, HH contribution to, 44, 44*t*
Antiretroviral therapy, CMV esophagitis treatment
        with, 31
Aorta arch anomalies, 83. *See also* Double aortic arch;
        Right-sided aortic arch
Ascorbic acid, pill-induced esophagitis caused by, 31
ASGE. *See* American Society for Gastrointestinal
        Endoscopy
Atherosclerosis, aorta abnormalities and, 83

Barrett's esophagus (BE)
    adenocarcinoma and, 65
    definition of, 52
    diagnosis, 52
    endoscopic findings and, 56
    endoscopic identification of, 52
    gastroesophageal reflux disease and prevalence of,
        58

HH presence and, 56, *56*
LES and, 52-54, *53*
long segment, 52, *53*
postfundoplication evaluation of, 79
short segment, 52, *52*
squamous epithelium, columnar epithelium
        tongues protruding into esophageal and,
        56, *57*
Barrett's metaplasia, 51-58
    adenocarcinoma, esophageal and, 56
    biopsy specimens of, dysplastic changes detected on,
        56-58
    chronic cough and, 3
    EGJ, mucosa migration above and, 22, 24
    LPR and, 3, 58
    screening recommendations for, 56
    survival rates, 58
BE. *See* Barrett's esophagus
Benzocaine, hypopharynx, 13
Biopsies, 90
Barrett's metaplasia, dysplastic changes detected by,
        56-58
    cup forceps for, 90
    herpes esophagitis diagnosed by, 31
    lesions, 90, *91*
    neoplasia, 60
    transnasal panendoscopy and, 90, *92*
Botulinum toxin type A
    achalasia treatment with, 77
    esophageal rings, A-type treated with, 38
Bravo delivery catheter, 101

Candida albicans, as esophagitis etiology, 26-30
Chronic cough
    Barrett's metaplasia and, 3
    TNE in patient's with, 2-3
Cirrhosis
    esophageal varices developed by, 74
    TNE examination of, 76
Clindamycin, pill-induced esophagitis caused by, 31
Clopidogrel bisulfate, 90
CMV. *See* Cytomegalovirus
Cytomegalovirus (CMV)
    as esophagitis etiology, 31
    glandular mucosa of stomach and, 31

103

DAA. *See* Double aortic arch
Decongestion, TNE and nasal, 11
Diaphragmatic hiatus, distal antireflux barrier and, 44
Diaphragmatic pinch, 54
Double aortic arch (DAA), 83
    esophagoscopic view of, *83*
Doxycycline, pill-induced esophagitis caused by, 31
Dysphagia, 26
    cause/site of, determining, 92, *93*
    esophageal neoplasms, malignant and, 64
    esophageal webs/rings causing, 38
    herpes esophagitis and resulting, 30-31
    posttherapy, 92
    Stevens-Johnson syndrome and, 85
    TNE evaluation of, 92, *93*
    tongue base endoscopic inspection and, 10, *10*
    vascular rings as cause of, 81
    vocal fold immobility in, 11, *11*
Dysphagia lusoria, *82*, 83
Dysplasia, postfundoplication evaluation of, 79

EE. *See* Eosinophilic esophagitis
EGD, transoral. *See* Esophagogastroduodenoscopy,
        transoral
EGJ. *See* Esophageal-gastric junction
Empiric acid, pill-induced esophagitis treatment with,
        32
Endoscope. *See also* American Society for
            Gastrointestinal Endoscopy
    BE and, 52, 56
    dysphagia, tongue base and inspection with, 10, *10*
    EE findings on, 34, *34*
    esophagitis appearance on
        Candida, 26, *29*
        caustic, *32, 33*
        CMV, 31
        reflux, 26
    HH evaluation with, 44
        sliding, 46, *49*
        type I, 46, *49*
    hypopharynx anatomy/technique and, 5-16
    nasal cavity anatomy/ technique and, 5-16
    PDL, 95
    postfundoplication evaluation with, 79
    tracheoesophageal fistula visualized with, *75*
    transoral, 19
EndoSheath, 12-13, *13*
Endosonography, submucosal lesion evaluation with,
        60
Eosinophilic esophagitis (EE), 34
    endoscopic findings of, 34, *34*
    presentation, 34
    treatment, 34
Epidermolysis bullosa dystrophica, 85
Epinephrine
    nasal cavity, 13
    TEP, 92, *93*

Epiphrenic diverticulum, 70
Esophageal adenocarcinoma, Barrett's metaplasia and,
        56
Esophageal cyst, 60
Esophageal dilation, 98-100
    hydrostatic balloon dilator for, 99, *99*
    Kelly clamp for, 98
    Savary dilators for, 98, *98*, 99
    stricture, severe, 100
    technique, 98-100, *99*
Esophageal disorders, miscellaneous, 69-87
    achalasia as, 77
    anastomotic evaluation and, 77
    epidermolysis bullosa dystrophica, 85
    esophageal diverticula as, 70-71
    esophageal foreign body as, 72, *73*
    esophageal manifestations of systemic diseases as, 84
    esophageal varices as, 74-76
    glycogenis acanthosis, 85, *86*
    mucosal bridges as, *86,* 87
    postfundoplication evaluation and, 79-81
    scleroderma as, 84
    Stevens-Johnson syndrome as, 85
    tracheoesophageal fistula as, 74
    vascular rings as, 81-83
Esophageal diverticula
    asymptomatic, 71, *71*
    classification of, 70
    diagnosis of, 71
    large, 71, 72
    postsurgical scarring and, 71, *71*
Esophageal foreign body
    rigid endoscopy treatment of, 72
    stomach advancement of, 72, *73, 74*
    technique for removal of, 72, 73
Esophageal manifestations of systemic disease, 84
Esophageal metaplasia/malignancy, LPR symptoms as
            indications of, 3
Esophageal neoplasms
    benign
        esophageal cyst as, 60
        fibrovascular polyp as, 61
        granular cell tumor as, 61
        hemangiomas as, 63, *63*
        inflammatory pseudotumor as, 63, *64*
        leiomyoma as, 60
        lipoma as, 61, *61*
        lymphangioma as, 63
        papilloma as, *62*, 63
    malignant
        adenocarcinoma, 65
        dysphagia and, 64
        squamous cell carcinoma as, 64
Esophageal rings, 37-40
    dysphagia caused by, 38
    lower
        A-ring as, 38, *39*
        B-ring as, 38, *39*

Esophageal stricture, 26, *29*

Esophageal ulcers
  adenocarcinoma and, 65, *67*
  Candida, 30, *30*
  CMV and, 31
  pill-induced, 32, *32*

Esophageal varices
  bleeding risk of, 74-76
  cirrhosis development of, 74
  TNE and appearance of, 76, *76*, 77

Esophageal webs, 37-40
  dysphagia caused by, 38
  proximal, 38, *40*

Esophageal-gastric junction (EGJ), *18*, 19
  Barrett's metaplasia and mucosa migration above,
      22, 24
  landmarks to identify, 19
  normal, 54, *55*
  SCJ proximity and, 56, *57*
  wrap location and, 79, *80*

Esophagitis, 25-34. *See also* Eosinophilic esophagitis
  BE and, 52
  Candida, 26-30
  endoscopic appearance of, 26, *29*
  histopathologic diagnosis of, 30
  mucosal plaques and, 26-30, *29*, 30
  risk factors for developing, 26
  symptoms, 26
  treatment, 30
  ulceration from, 30, *30*
  caustic, 32-34
    acid injury as cause of, 33
    alkali injury as cause of, 32, 33
    endoscopic appearance of, 32
    endoscopic evaluation of, 33
    esophagoscopic evaluation of, 33-34
    first-degree burns from, 32
    management, long-term of, 34
    management of, 33
    second-degree burns from, 32
    stricture/stenosis resulting from, 32
    third-degree burns from, 32
  CMV, 31
    diagnosis, 31
    endoscopic features of, 31
    esophageal ulcers and, 31
    symptoms, 31
    treatment, 31
  etiologies, 26
  herpes, 30-31
    biopsy and diagnosis, 31
    dysphagia resulting from, 30-31
    symptoms, presenting of, 30
    treating, 31
  LA classification system for, 26
  pill-induced, 31-32
    antibiotics-causing, 31
    cause of, 31

etiology of injury and, 31
  treatment for, 32
  ulcerated, 32, *32*
reflux, 26
  chronic, 26, *29*
  endoscopic findings for, 26
  grade A, 26, *27*
  grade B, 26, *27*
  grade C, 26, *28*
  grade D, 26, *28*
  pH testing and, 100
  stricture and, 26, *29*

Esophagogastroduodenoscopy (EGD), transoral
    gastrointestinal oral endoscopy appliance for, 9, *9*
  image orientation on video monitor for, 6, *7*

Esophagoscope
  caustic esophagitis evaluated by, 33-34
  DAA viewed with, 83, *83*
  holding, 14, *14*
  rigid, 19
  tracheoesophageal fistula visualized with, 75

Esophagus. *See also* Barrett's esophagus; Esophagitis;
      Lower esophageal sphincter; Upper
      esophageal sphincter
  anatomy, 18
  deviation of, 19
  external compressions, 19, *19*
    aortic, 19, *19, 20*
    diaphragmatic compression, 19, *19, 20*
    left mainstem bronchus, 19, *19, 20*
  heterotopic gastric mucosa seen in, 24, *24*
  length, 18
  obstruction, 72
  squamous epithelium-lined, 18, 19
  TNE esophagoscope insertion into, 14-15, *15*
  TNE visualization of, 19

Fibrovascular polyp, 61
Fluconazole, *Candida* esophagitis treatment with, 30
Fluticasone propionate, EE treatment with, 34
Foscarnet, CMV esophagitis treatment with, 31
Fundoplication. *See also* Postfundoplication evalua-
      tion
  complications after, 79
  goals of, 79
  intact, 81, *81*
  integrity evaluation for, 79
  slipped, 79, *80, 82*
  wrap zone, 79

Ganciclovir, CMV esophagitis treatment with, 31
Gastric rugae, HH and, *22*, 24
Gastroesophageal reflux disease
  BE prevalence and, 58
  Schatzki's ring and, 38
Gastroesophageal variceal bleeding, 74

Gastroscope, per-oral, 11-12
Gel-Cap technique, 93
Glandular mucosa, CMV and stomach, 31
Glycogenic acanthosis, 85, *86*
Granular cell tumor, 61

Hemangiomas, 63, *63*
Hemorrhage, variceal, 76
Herpes, as esophagitis etiology, 30-31
Heterotopic gastric mucosa, esophagus and, 24, *24*
HH. *See* Hiatal hernia
Hiatal hernia (HH), 43-50
  age and prevalence of, 44
  BE and presence of, 56, *56*
  endoscopic evaluation of, 44
  gastric rugae and, *22, 24*
  hiatus location and, 46
  lax diaphragmatic crura and retroflexion view of, *23, 24*
  mixed, 46-50, *48*
    retroflexion evaluation of, 50
  paraesophageal, 46, *48*
  reflux promoted by, 44, 44*t*
  rugae proximal migration and, 46, *46*
  SCJ location and, 54, *55*
  sliding, 46, *47*
    endoscopic diagnosis of, 46, *49*
  type I, 46, *47*
    endoscopic diagnosis of, 46, *49*
  type II, 46, *48*
  type III, 46-50, *48*
    retroflexion evaluation of, 50
Hiatus, 46, *46*
His angle-created valve effect, distal antireflux barrier and, 44, *45*
Hydrostatic balloon dilator, for esophageal dilation, 99, *99*
Hypopharyngeal diverticulum, 70, *70*
Hypopharynx
  anesthesia for, 13
  EGD, transoral video monitor image orientation of, 6, *7*
  endoscopic anatomy of, technique and, 5-16
  stricture/stenosis resulting from caustic esophagitis in, 32, *33*

Inflammatory pseudotumor, 63, *64*
Intraluminal tumors, benign, 61

Kelly clamp, for esophageal dilation, 98

LA classification system. *See* Los Angeles classification system

Laryngeal examination, patient acceptance/tolerance, 16
Laryngeal lesions, 10, *11*
  PDL management of, 93
Laryngopharyngeal reflux (LPR)
  Barrett's metaplasia in persons with, 3, 58
  esophageal metaplasia/malignancy indicated by, 3
  screening and, 3
  TNE indications for patients with, 3
Lax diaphragmatic crura, HH seen during retroflexion view and, *23,* 24
Leiomyoma, 60
LES. *See* Lower esophageal sphincter
Lesions
  biopsies of, 90, *91*
  laryngeal, 10, *11,* 93
  neoplasia and size of, 60
  submucosal, endosonography evaluation of, 60
Lidocaine
  maximal dose for, 90
  nasal cavity, 13
  PDL and, 97
  TEP, 92, 93
  TNE and, 90
Lipoma, 61, *61*
Los Angeles (LA) classification system, 26
Lower esophageal sphincter (LES)
  achalasia as relaxation failure of, 77
  anatomy, 18
  BE and, 52-54, *53*
  high-pressure zone in, 44, *45*
  intrinsic, distal antireflux barrier and, 44, *45*
  proximal border of, 46, *47*
  TNE and transversing, 15
  visualizing, 15
Lymphangioma, 63

Midesophageal diverticulum, 70
Mucosal bridges, *86,* 87
Mucosal plaques, Candida esophagitis and, 26-30, *29, 30*

Nasal cavity
  anatomy, 6-11
    nasopharynx and, 10, *10*
    scope in, passing through and, *8,* 8-9, *9*
    TNE and, 6
    variations in, *8,* 8-9, *9*
  anesthesia, 11, 13
  endoscopic anatomy of, technique and, 5-16
  scope in, passing through, 6-8, 6-9
  structures, primary visualized in, 6, *7*
  TNE and vasoconstriction in, 6
  vasoconstriction, 6, 13
Nasal patency, 90
Nasal polyps, 9, *9*

Nasal septal deviations, 8, *8*
Nasal septal perforation, *8*, 8-9
Nasopharynx, 10, *10*
  stricture/stenosis resulting from caustic esophagitis
    in, 32, *33*
Neoplasia, 59-67
  biopsy, 60
  esophageal neoplasms as
    benign, 60-63
    malignant, 64-65
  lesion size and, 60
  survival and detection of, 60
Nystatin, *Candida* esophagitis treatment with, 30

Odynophagia, 26
Ora serrata, 18, *18*
Oxymetazoline
  nasal cavity, 13
  PDL and, 97

Papilloma, *62*, 63
  PDL treatment of large, *96*, 97, *97*
Paterson-Kelly syndrome, esophageal webs and, 38
Patient acceptance/tolerance, laryngeal
    examination/TNE, 16
PDL. *See* Pulsed-dye laser
pH probes, placement
  ambulatory, 100
  hard-wired, 100
  TNE for, *100*, 100-101
  wireless, 100
    Bravo delivery catheter for, 101
Plummer-Vinson syndrome, esophageal webs and, 38
Postfundoplication evaluation, 79-81
  BE, 79
  dysplasia, 79
  endoscopic, 79
Potassium chloride, pill-induced esophagitis caused
    by, 31
Procedures, 89-101
  biopsies, 92
  esophageal dilation, 98-100
  office-based, 90
  PDL, 93-97
  pH probes, placement of as, 100-101
  posttherapy dysphagia, 92
  tracheoesophageal puncture, 92-93
Pulsed-dye laser (PDL), 93-97
  anesthesia for, 97
  cancer therapy and, 95
  endoscope required for, 95
  indications, 95
  laryngeal lesions managed by, 93
  papilloma treatment with, *96*, 97, *97*
  safety precautions for, 97
  technique for, *96*, 97

Quinidine, pill-induced esophagitis caused by, 31

RAA. *See* Right-sided aortic arch
Raynaud's phenomenon, 84
Retroflexion, type II HH evaluated with, 50
Right subclavian artery (RSCA), 83
Right-sided aortic arch (RAA), 83
Rigid endoscopy, 72
RSCA. *See* Right subclavian artery

Savary dilators, for esophageal dilation, 98, *98, 99*
Schatzki's ring, 38, *39*
SCJ. *See* Squamocolumnar junction
Scleroderma, 84, *84*
Squamocolumnar junction (SCJ), 18, *18*
  BE and, 52
  circumference, 46
  EGJ and proximity of, 56, *57*
  irregular, 19-24, *21*
  location, HH and, 54, *55*
  normal, 54, *54*
  retroverted view of, *23*, 24
  TNE and transversing, 15
  visualizing, 15
Squamous cell carcinoma, 64
  advanced, 64, *65*
  esophageal mucosa changes and, 64, *66*
Squamous epithelium, 18, 19
  columnar epithelium tongues protruding into
    esophageal, 56, *57*
Squamous papilloma, *62*, 63
Stenosis, caustic esophagitis resulting in, 32
Steroids, epidermolysis bullosa dystrophica treatment
    with, 85
Stevens-Johnson syndrome, 85, *85*
Stomach, suctioning, 15
Stricture
  caustic esophagitis resulting in, 32
  esophageal, 26, *29*
  esophageal dilation for patients with severe, 100

TEP. *See* Tracheoesophageal puncture
Tetracycline, pill-induced esophagitis caused by, 31
TNE. *See* Transnasal esophagoscopy
Tongue base, dysphagia and endoscopic inspection of,
    10, *10*
Torus tubarius, 10, *10*
Tracheoesophageal fistula
  diagnosis, 74
  endoscopic/esophagoscopic view of, *75*
  etiologies, 74
  scalpel opening of, 93, *94*
Tracheoesophageal puncture (TEP), 92-93
  anesthetics, 92-93
  Gel-Cap technique for, 93

Tracheoesophageal puncture (TEP) *(continued)*
   needle for, 93, *94*
   prosthesis placement for, 93, *95*
   secondary, 92-93
   TNE for, 92
Transnasal esophagoscopy (TNE)
   anesthesia, topical for, 6, *6*, 11, 90
      techniques for delivering, 90
   chronic cough, 2-3
   cirrhotic patient examination with, 76
   decongestion for, 11
   dysphagia evaluated with, 92, *93*
   early, warning signs for, 2
   esophageal mucosa visualization during, 15-16
   esophageal varices appearance on, 76, *76*, *77*
   esophagitis found during, 26
   esophagoscope size for, 12
   esophagus and inserting esophagoscope for, 14-15,
      15
   esophagus visualized during, 19
   fiberoptic add-on camera, *12*
      EndoSheath and, 12-13, *13*
   fishing-pole technique for holding esophagoscope
      for, 14, *14*
   head and neck cancer use of, 90
   indications for, 1-3
      diagnostic, 2
      esophageal, 2, *2t*
      extraesophageal, 2, *3t*
      LPR and, 3
      therapeutic, 2
   LES and, 15
   nasal cavity anatomy and, 6
   normal, 17-24
   patient acceptance/tolerance of, 16
   patient selection for, 90
   pH probe placement and, *100*, 100-101
   postcricoid visualization during, 16
   SCJ and, 15
   standard technique for holding esophagoscope for,
      14, *14*
   suture line after hypopharyngeal/gastroesophageal
      surgery assessed with, 77, *78*
   technique, 11-16
   TEP, 92
   UES transversal and, 15
   vasoconstriction in nasal cavity and, 6
   video chip flexible endoscope system, 12, *12*
Transnasal panendoscopy, biopsy and, 90, *92*

UES. *See* Upper esophageal sphincter
Ultrathin endoscopy, 76
Upper esophageal sphincter (UES)
   anatomy, 18
   TNE and traversing, 15

Vascular rings, 81-82
   DAA as cause of complete, 83
   diagnosis of, 81-83, *83*
video-assisted thorascopic surgery for, 83
Vasoconstriction, nasal cavity, 6, 13
Video-assisted thorascopic surgery, 83
Vocal fold motion abnormalities (paralysis/paresis),
   10-11, *11*

Warfarin, 90

Zenker's diverticulum, 70, *70*
Z-line, 18, *18*
   irregular, 19-24, *21*
   location, 54